KETO SMOOTHIE RECIPE BOOK

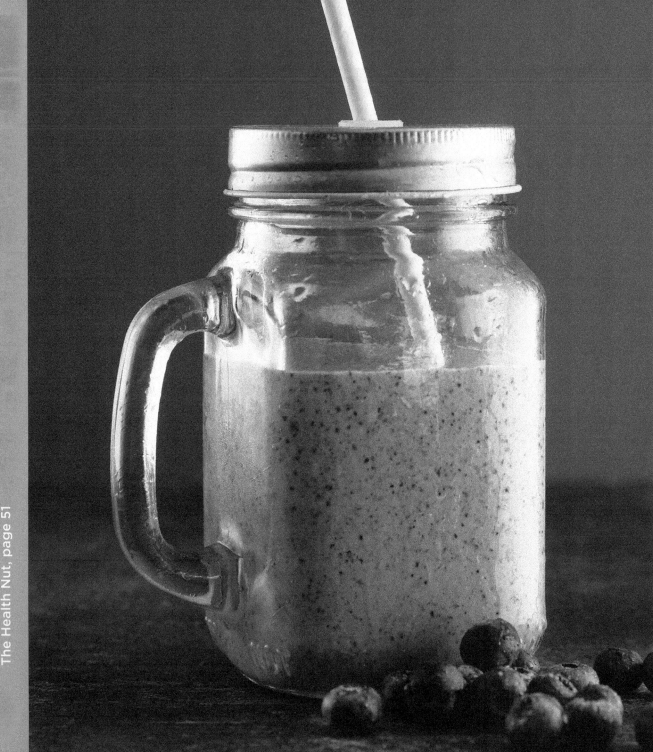

The Health Nut, page 51

KETO SMOOTHIE
RECIPE BOOK

75 High-Fat, Low-Carb Smoothies and Shakes

Tasha Metcalf

**ROCKRIDGE
PRESS**

For my little chefs, Sebina and Felix

For general information on our other products and services or to obtain technical support, please contact our Customer Care Department within the United States at (866) 744-2665, or outside the United States at (510) 253-0500.

Rockridge Press publishes its books in a variety of electronic and print formats. Some content that appears in print may not be available in electronic books, and vice versa.

TRADEMARKS: Rockridge Press and the Rockridge Press logo are trademarks or registered trademarks of Callisto Media Inc. and/or its affiliates, in the United States and other countries, and may not be used without written permission. All other trademarks are the property of their respective owners. Rockridge Press is not associated with any product or vendor mentioned in this book.

Interior and Cover Designer: Jill Lee
Art Producer: Megan Baggott
Editor: Anna Pulley
Production Editor: Dylan Julian
Production Manager: Lanore Coloprisco

Cover photo, Elena Veselova/StockFood USA; Mathias Neubauer/Gräfe & Unzer Verlag/StockFood USA, ii; Fanny Rådvik/StockFood USA, vii; Jörn Rynio/Gräfe & Unzer Verlag/StockFood USA, viii; Kati Finell/StockFood USA, 15; Sporrer/Skowronek/StockFood USA, 16; Jan Wischnewski/StockFood USA, 34; Jill Chen/Stocksy United, 53; Ian Garlick/StockFood USA, 54; Babett Lupaneszku/Stocksy United, 72; Jan Wischnewski/StockFood USA, 90; Trinette Reed/Stocksy United, 107

Paperback ISBN: 978-1-63878-353-4
eBook ISBN: 978-1-63878-578-1
R0

CONTENTS

INTRODUCTION

Welcome to the *Keto Smoothie Recipe Book*! I'm Tasha, and I'm going to teach you how to enjoy smoothies without relying on carbs for flavor and energy. By the time you've finished reading this book, you'll have an arsenal of delicious recipes that fit your macros. You'll also know which ingredients to stock your pantry with (and which to pass on) and be lifelong BFFs with your blender. More than anything, I hope you come away from this book with the mindset that keto can be easy—it doesn't have to feel complicated, overwhelming, or restrictive.

I wish this book existed when I made the switch to low-carb living many years ago. Prompted by my healthcare practitioner, I transitioned to a therapeutic ketogenic diet to manage my polycystic ovary syndrome (PCOS) symptoms, but I felt clueless in the beginning. Lost and confused about what foods to eat, I turned to the internet for help. There were so few resources available back then; when I tried to find keto-friendly recipes, the ones I found were time-consuming and required elaborate cooking and baking skills or expensive tools that I didn't own. I've always loved cooking, but who has the time to spend hours in the kitchen every day? I needed practical recipes that I could use on busy days to successfully change my eating habits. Rather than give up, I started to make my own quick and easy recipes. Eventually, I started sharing them. It turns out other people needed convenient recipes, too!

Smoothies have always been a go-to way for me to start my day, but when I started keto, I initially retired them from my menu. I assumed, based on the high-carb milk, syrups, honey, and high-sugar fruits I was using, that smoothies were off-limits. *Oh, how wrong I was!* Over the years, I've developed so many amazing recipes after experimenting with more unconventional, keto-friendly ingredients. Smoothies and shakes have become an integral part of my health journey and continue to play an important role in my nutrition plan today. I'm eager to show you how so you can benefit from them as well.

For me, the most rewarding part of developing keto recipes is challenging the restrictive mindset that is so common in diet culture. Changing my perception from

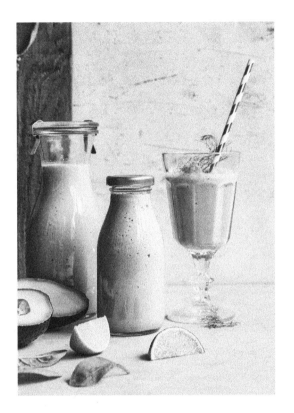

"I can't eat that anymore" to "Let's try this ingredient instead" was a total game-changer. There were so many new, healthier ways to enjoy my favorite meals and comfort foods (my beloved smoothies included) without feeling like I was missing out. To that end, I hope to highlight the many wonderful, nutrient-dense ingredients we can enjoy on keto and focus less on what we "can't" have.

Since starting on my own health journey, I've become a certified nutritionist, completing a master's degree in human nutrition and diving deep into the research to help others use food as medicine to heal. I now specialize in low-carb ketogenic dietary patterns to help others who are struggling as I did. In addition to working with nutrition clients in my private practice, I've also written several books about the keto diet, and I teach wellness workshops and develop recipes and meal plans for Ketogasm.com. My personal mission is to help make keto easy and sustainable; that's why I'm so happy to share this comprehensive resource to help simplify your path to health and wellness.

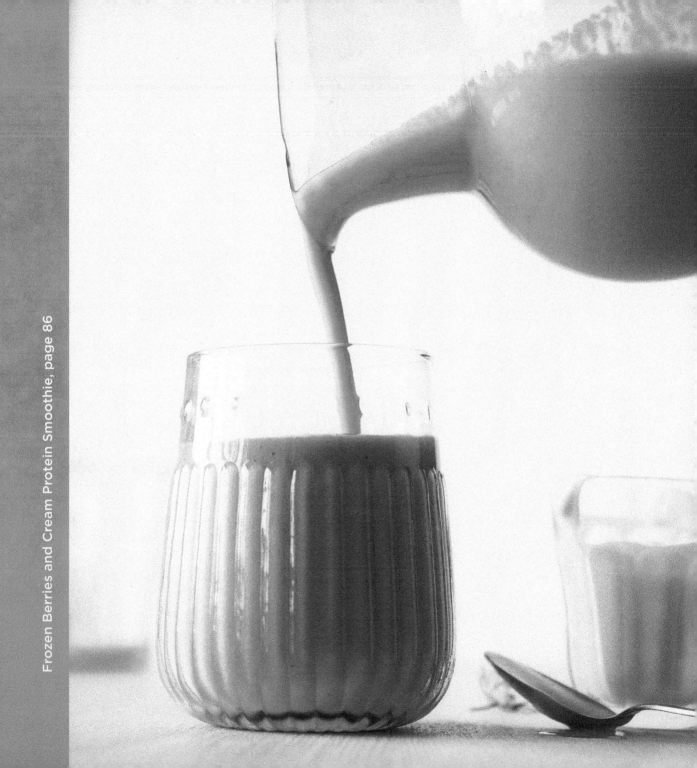

Frozen Berries and Cream Protein Smoothie, page 86

CHAPTER 1

KETO
SMOOTHIE BASICS

To kick things off, we'll review the nutritional basics of keto to ensure you're on the right track. First, we'll brush up on our knowledge of ketosis and macronutrients, including which carbs to count toward your daily total. You'll also find tips to help you feel your best as you transition away from a high-carb diet. Next, we'll jump into the ins and outs of smoothie making, including which ingredients to stock up on, what blender to use, and how to get the perfect smoothie every time.

The Keto Diet

Keto (short for "ketogenic") is a dietary pattern that relies on carb restriction to induce ketosis. The body prefers to burn carbs, so by depriving your body of these carbs, you can shift your metabolism and direct the body to produce ketones and burn fat for energy instead of sugar from carbs. Getting into ketosis usually takes a few days of very low-carb eating. When you initially limit carbs from your diet, the body must first burn through stored sugars in your liver and muscles (glycogen) before ramping up ketone production and fat metabolism. Eventually, the body becomes more efficient at using ketones and burning fat for energy—this is ketosis. This increased efficiency is also known as fat adaptation, which often results in boosted energy, mood, and appetite regulation.

Macronutrients

Macronutrients ("macros," for short) are the nutrients that your body needs in the largest amounts: fats, proteins, and carbs. These nutrients are the building blocks of food that supply the body with fuel to burn for energy. They also support various bodily functions and structures. Keto relies on optimizing macronutrient ratios to support ketosis and burn fat as the primary fuel source. This typically requires low-carb, high-fat food intake, and individual macro targets depend on body composition, activity levels, and health goals.

Fat: 60 to 90 percent. Fat provides 9 calories per gram, making it the most energy-dense macronutrient. Most high-carb dietary patterns call for reduced fat intake to balance or reduce calories. However, the reverse is true for keto! When carbs are restricted, the largest source of energy becomes fat. In keto, dietary fat typically makes up the biggest portion of your daily calorie intake. Fatty acids, like those found in foods rich in omega-3s and omega-6s, can also convert to ketones for fuel. Fat is vital for absorbing vitamins and minerals and producing hormones, essential molecules, and structures throughout the body. It also adds texture and rich flavor to foods.

Protein: 10 to 30 percent. Protein provides 4 calories per gram, though it is not typically a primary fuel source. Instead, it provides amino acid building blocks to maintain lean body mass and synthesize new compounds. Eating adequate protein is key to preserving muscle mass, especially when dieting. Protein is the most satiating macro, helping you feel full. During ketosis, amino acids also support glucose production that stabilizes blood sugar; additionally, they fuel cells that cannot use fat or ketones for fuel. Individual protein needs vary, with active individuals requiring higher levels.

Carbs: 4 to 19 percent. Carbohydrates provide 4 calories per gram, though intake is limited on a keto diet. Carb restriction induces ketosis, forcing the body to burn fat as a primary fuel source. Most keto dieters keep their daily carb intake below 50 grams total. Carbohydrates are not the primary source of energy on keto; rather, acceptable carb sources provide vitamins, minerals, phytonutrients, and fiber critical for health.

CARBS VERSUS NET CARBS

Dietary sources of carbohydrates include sugar, starches, and fiber components from food. Sugar alcohols also fall under the carb category. They each impact the body differently. Sugars and starches negatively impact ketosis by reducing fat burning and ketone production. Fiber and sugar alcohols are not metabolized the same way. Our bodies cannot directly digest fiber; insoluble fibers pass through the digestive tract as unabsorbed roughage, while gut bacteria ferment soluble fibers (great for the microbiome!). Sugar alcohols are similar in that they aren't metabolized and used for energy. As a result, neither of these components directly impacts ketosis. For that reason, many people subtract fiber and sugar alcohols from the total carbs to yield "net carbs." Net carbs are the carbs that the body metabolizes and uses for energy—the ones that can influence ketosis. On average, net carbs end up being 20 to 30 grams per day.

Embarking on Your Keto Journey

When you first start a keto diet, side effects may occur, depending on how you previously ate. The transition tends to be relatively smooth with minimal side effects if you come from a low-carb dietary pattern, because your body is less reliant on sugar for fuel and has already made adaptations to thrive on low-carb intake. However, if you typically eat a high-carb diet and suddenly cut most of the carbs out, your body has to make several adjustments to switch from burning sugar to burning fat. During this process, you may experience some discomfort and flulike symptoms, known as keto flu. Common symptoms include headache, nausea, cramping, irritability, light-headedness, lack of energy, and tiredness.

Dehydration and electrolyte imbalance are responsible for these symptoms. When you drop carbs from your diet, your body rapidly burns through stored carbs in your muscles and liver, depleting water stores and electrolytes in the process. You can prevent these symptoms by staying hydrated and eating electrolyte-rich foods. The recipes in chapter 2 will help you with this.

Smoothies: The Key to Keto

Smoothies and shakes are a must in my meal planning and recipe tool kit. Endless flavor combinations satisfy cravings, whether sweet, savory, cold, warm, fruity, nutty, or chocolaty—you name it. The variety and fun flavors make sticking with your health goals enjoyable, and the press-of-a-button meal prep feels effortless. Since you can mix in so many different ingredients, smoothies provide a unique opportunity to boost your nutrition with nuts, seeds, fruits, veggies, or even dietary supplements.

Smoothies and shakes also have keto-specific benefits.

They restore electrolyte levels. Smoothies made with nutrient-dense, whole-food ingredients provide electrolytes needed to ward off keto flu and thrive while eating low-carb.

They provide an easy way to get an extra shot of fat or protein. You can easily adjust smoothies to fit your personal macro goals by adding extra protein or fat to support physical activity, energy needs, and body composition goals.

They simplify meal prep. Convenience is the secret to sustainability and success. Shakes and smoothies can't get any easier—press a button, and meals are ready!

They can deliver dietary supplements. Powdered and oil-based supplements enable you to supercharge your nutrition. Electrolytes, collagen, fish oil, MCT oil, and protein powder are just a few smoothie add-ins.

The Blender

The blender is the keystone of smoothie making. For smoothie success, the blender must be able to handle both liquids and challenging solid ingredients, crush through ice cubes, break down frozen fruits, and cut through fibrous, stringy produce (looking at you, celery!). You also need a machine that can tolerate routine usage, making high-power motors a desirable feature for daily use. Consider whether you will be making smoothies for one person or a larger group.

The following blenders are the best options for smoothie making.

Immersion or stick blenders. Handheld immersion blenders are thin tools that fit directly into a cup or bowl containing smoothie ingredients, making them an excellent space-saving option. You can use them in both small and large containers, helpful for scaling recipes up. The immersion blender is best used for smoothies with soft ingredients; ice and frozen foods may be overpowering to the small blades and motor.

Single-serving or bullet blenders. These small blenders with a mixing container that often doubles as the serving cup are perfect for smoothie making for one.

Countertop or commercial blenders. If you're serious about smoothie making, I recommend investing in a countertop blender with a high-power motor. Though there are budget-friendly options, the price range tops out higher in this category with tools designed for commercial use. These blenders can tackle even the toughest ingredients and are more likely to survive daily use.

Smoothie Ingredients

You may be surprised to learn how many ingredients are keto-friendly, but don't feel like you need to run out and gather all the items listed here. Build out your smoothie pantry over time and keep your go-to ingredients stocked so your favorite smoothie is just minutes away. When selecting new products, always opt for unsweetened versions.

Dairy

Lactose is the natural sugar found in dairy. Cow's milk is especially high in lactose, making it difficult to fit within keto-friendly macros as a full drink or smoothie base. Lower-carb dairy options include:

- Butter
- Cheeses, hard and soft, such as cream cheese, provolone, asiago, gorgonzola, mozzarella, Manchego, Swiss, goat, cheddar, Parmesan, mascarpone, brie, Gruyère, ricotta, feta, and cottage cheese
- Ghee
- Heavy (whipping) cream
- Plain Greek yogurt

Fats and Oils

Oils and fats provide additional energy and a rich, creamy texture to smoothies. Healthy fat sources are antioxidant and anti-inflammatory and help the body absorb vitamins and minerals. Medium-chain triglycerides (MCTs) are quick-digesting fats that provide rapid energy and enhance ketone production. MCT oil is wonderful for smoothies since it's pourable and has a neutral flavor. These fats include:

- Avocado oil
- Butter
- Coconut oil
- Extra-virgin olive oil
- Ghee
- MCT oil

Dairy-Free Milks and Yogurts

Dairy-free milks are low in carbs and make excellent liquid bases for smoothies and shakes; yogurts thicken them. Read nutrition labels and ingredient lists to avoid added sugars and starches. I recommend:

- Coconut milk and coconut milk beverage*, cream, and yogurt
- Nut milks, including almond, cashew**, hazelnut, macadamia nut, and walnut milk
- Pea protein milk
- Seed milk, such as flaxseed, hemp seed, sesame, and sunflower milk
- Soy milk and yogurt

*Coconut milk beverage is different from coconut milk. The beverage can be found in the refrigerated section by the dairy and refrigerated nondairy milk options and near other nondairy pantry items. Delicious and Pacific Foods are two popular brands.

**Store-bought cashew milk is fine; homemade may be higher in carbs.

Nuts, Seeds, and Plant-Based Butters

Except cashews, most nuts and seeds (and nut and seed butters) are high in fiber and relatively low in net carbs, fitting keto macros within moderation. Some options include:

- Nuts and nut butters, including almonds, brazil nuts, hazelnuts, macadamia nuts, peanuts, pecans, pine nuts, pistachios, and walnuts
- Seeds and seed butters, including chia seeds, flaxseed, hemp seed, sesame seeds (tahini), pumpkin seeds, and sunflower seeds

Fruits

Many fruits are high in natural sugar, making them tricky to incorporate into a keto diet. Avoid dried fruit, canned fruit, and commercial fruit juices or concentrates—all are high in sugar. Instead, try lower-carb options like:

- Berries, including blackberries, blueberries, boysenberries, raspberries, and strawberries
- Citrus, including grapefruit, lemons, limes, and oranges (freshly squeezed citrus juices can be used in small quantities but are too high in carbs to use as a smoothie base)
- Savory fruits, including avocado, coconut, olives, pumpkin, tomatillos, and tomatoes

Vegetables and Fresh Herbs

Leafy greens, non-starchy vegetables, and fresh herbs are low in carbohydrates, jam-packed with nutrients, and hands down my favorite smoothie ingredients. Smoothies make it easy to sneak in foods for their nutritional benefit and mask the taste with other ingredients. Avoid super-starchy vegetables—potatoes, yams, yucca—to keep carbs low. I recommend:

- Green leafy veggies, including arugula, beet greens, bok choy, dandelion greens, kale, mustard greens, romaine lettuce, spinach, Swiss chard, and watercress
- Herbs, including basil, chives, cilantro, dill, lemongrass, oregano, parsley, peppermint, spearmint, tarragon, and thyme
- Non-starchy vegetables, including asparagus, banana pepper, bell pepper, broccoli, carrots, cauliflower, celery, chayote squash, cucumbers, jicama, microgreens, mushrooms, pickles, radishes, rhubarb, sprouts, and zucchini
- Sea vegetables, including chlorella, dulse, kelp, nori, and spirulina

Chocolate and Cocoa Powder

Dark chocolate consists primarily of cocoa and has less sugar than milk chocolate. Typically, the darker the chocolate, the fewer the carbs. Some brands, like Lily's and ChocZero, specialize in chocolate of all kinds, made with keto-friendly sweeteners. Try:

- 80 percent or higher dark chocolate
- Cacao nibs
- Cocoa butter
- Cocoa powder

Salt, Spices, and Extracts

Seasonings can transform a bland dish into something delightful. Spices are used in small amounts, keeping carbs low and boosting the flavor of your keto smoothies. Some spice blends may contain sugar, so read nutrition labels on commercial spice mixes. Salts balance flavors and bump up the sodium content, and salt alternatives boost potassium and electrolytes. Extracts deliver natural flavors as a swap for high-carb ingredients. Some suggestions are:

- Extracts, including almond, anise, banana, mango, maple, mint, orange, peach, pineapple, raspberry, strawberry, vanilla, and watermelon
- Salt, including Celtic salt, Himalayan pink or black salt, Kosher salt, red or black Hawaiian salt, sea salt, and table salt

- Salt alternatives: potassium chloride, such as Morton Lite Salt, NoSalt, and Nu Salt
- Spices, including allspice, caraway seed, cardamom, cayenne pepper, chili powder, cinnamon, cloves, coriander seed, cumin, curry powder, fennel seed, garlic, ginger, mace, mustard seed, nutmeg, onion powder, paprika, pepper, pumpkin pie spice, turmeric powder, and vanilla bean

Coffee and Tea

Coffee and tea provide a liquid smoothie base that is nearly carb-free. Just allow them to cool before mixing into cold smoothies. Any plain coffee or tea will do, but watch out for high-carb additives in pre-brewed options or blended mixes. Some options are:

- Coffee, including black coffee, cold brew, espresso, and instant coffee
- Herbal tea, including anise seed, chamomile, cinnamon, dandelion, elderberry, ginger, hibiscus, hibiscus flower, honeybush, jasmine, lavender, lemongrass, licorice, peppermint, raspberry leaf, rooibos, rosehip, rosemary, turmeric, and yerba mate
- Non-herbal tea, including black, green, matcha powder, and oolong

PROTEIN POWDER AND SWEETENERS

Protein powders offer a convenient way to boost the protein content of smoothies. This can help you hit your protein macro, support muscle recovery after a workout, and make the drink more filling. However, many flavored protein powders rely on high-carb ingredients and sweeteners. Unflavored protein powder supplements for smoothies tend to be lower in carbs, and the neutral taste prevents competing flavors. Whey protein isolate and egg white protein powder are popular options for keto; my personal favorites are TGS and Jay Robb brands, respectively. Collagen hydrolysate powder is a supplemental protein source that supports musculoskeletal and skin health. Plant-based options include soy, pea, and rice protein isolates. If you prefer flavored protein powders, check the nutrition label to ensure that your choice is low in carbs (less than 4 grams per serving) and uses keto-friendly sweeteners.

Yes, you can have sweeteners on keto! Sugar alcohols don't directly impact ketosis. Keto-friendly sweeteners include erythritol, stevia, monkfruit, and allulose. These don't necessarily swap out in a 1:1 ratio. Compared to regular sugar, erythritol and allulose are slightly less sweet; stevia and monkfruit are much sweeter than the real deal. Allulose and monkfruit blends are my favorites because they don't have a weird aftertaste.

Smoothie Making 101

Making smoothies is straightforward, but I have a foolproof method to get you the perfect blend every time. Whether you want a more pourable texture or prefer it so thick that a spoon stands up in it, the ideal smoothie is *smooth*. You don't want clumps, gritty powders, or surprise ice shards that require you to chew your drink. The key to achieving this comes down to the order in which things are added to the blender. As a rule, liquids go first, followed by powders, produce, and ice.

Step 1: Liquids. In a blender, combine the base liquid and any other fluids used in smaller quantities for flavoring or nutrition content—for example, an almond milk base with MCT oil or a coconut cream base with vanilla extract. For the sake of smoothie making, think of yogurts and nut butters as liquids.

Step 2: Powders. Next, add any powdery or granulated ingredients—anything that might puff up into a cloud of dust. This includes seasonings, spices, salt, protein powders, and certain supplements. You want these ingredients to have contact with the liquids and blender blades so they can incorporate into the mixture. When these types of ingredients sit on top, they often coat the blender lid instead of mixing into the smoothie.

Step 3: Produce. Bulkier ingredients are added next: nuts, seeds, fruits, vegetables, and so on. The secret to achieving a super-thick texture is using frozen ingredients.

Step 4: Blend. Let the blender focus on blending. Save the ice crushing for later. This allows all the ingredients to get chopped, liquified, and incorporated without ice interference. Adjust the blender speed to accommodate the ingredients: Liquids and soft foods can blend at low speeds; hard and frozen items require higher speed.

Step 5: Scrape and test. After blending, inspect for any ingredients stuck to the sides and scrape them down into the mixture. Test the consistency and make adjustments. Too thick? Adding more base liquid or water will thin it out. Too thin? Adding ice will thicken it up.

Step 6: Ice. Optionally, add ice to the blender for a thick, frosty blended drink. Use the ice crush setting on the blender.

INSTANT SMOOTHIES

My favorite thing about smoothies and shakes is how effortless they are to prepare. Can it get any easier? Actually, it can! Instead of measuring individual ingredients each time you make a smoothie, consider prepping "smoothie packs" for the freezer. That way, everything is ready to go straight into the blender whenever the mood hits.

To make a smoothie pack:

1. Label a freezer-safe container with the recipe name, date, and liquid to be added.
2. Gather all the ingredients except for the base liquid. Small liquid quantities used for flavor are fine to include.
3. Measure out the ingredients and add them to the container, seal, and pop in the freezer.
4. When you're ready to blend, combine the base liquid and frozen ingredients in a blender and blend until smooth.

About the Recipes

The recipes in this book are organized by theme to help you quickly find the recipe that suits your needs and cravings. Chapter 2 kicks us off with smoothies that hydrate and restore. These recipes are great for anyone doing keto, but athletes and people just getting started on keto may find them especially helpful to ward off keto flu. Chapter 3 focuses on smoothies using nuts, seeds, and their butters in tasty and inventive ways. Chapter 4 is all about decadent, dessertlike smoothies that will make you forget all about sugar-filled treats. Chapter 5 focuses on fruity smoothies and will help you navigate the confusing terrain of keto-friendly fruits with ease. Chapter 6 is filled with savory smoothie recipes that will nourish your body and delight your palate with surprising flavor combinations.

Every recipe has been developed to stay within keto nutritional parameters. Most recipes contain at least 20 grams of fat and no more than 15 grams of net carbs (though many are much lower). The recipes are in order from lowest to highest net carbs. Protein content varies but can be boosted with protein powders as needed. Each recipe also provides calculated nutrition information, including calories, protein, fat, total carbs, fiber, net carbs, sugar alcohols, and macronutrient ratios.

Additionally, you'll find the following nutrition-specific recipe labels:

High Fat: 30 grams or more per serving

High Protein: 20 grams or more per serving

Super Low Carb: Less than 10 grams of net carbs per serving

Net Carbs: Total carbs − fiber − erythritol (sugar alcohols)

Finally, the recipes include tips for variations, with simple additions or swaps to change up the flavor. Now let's get blending!

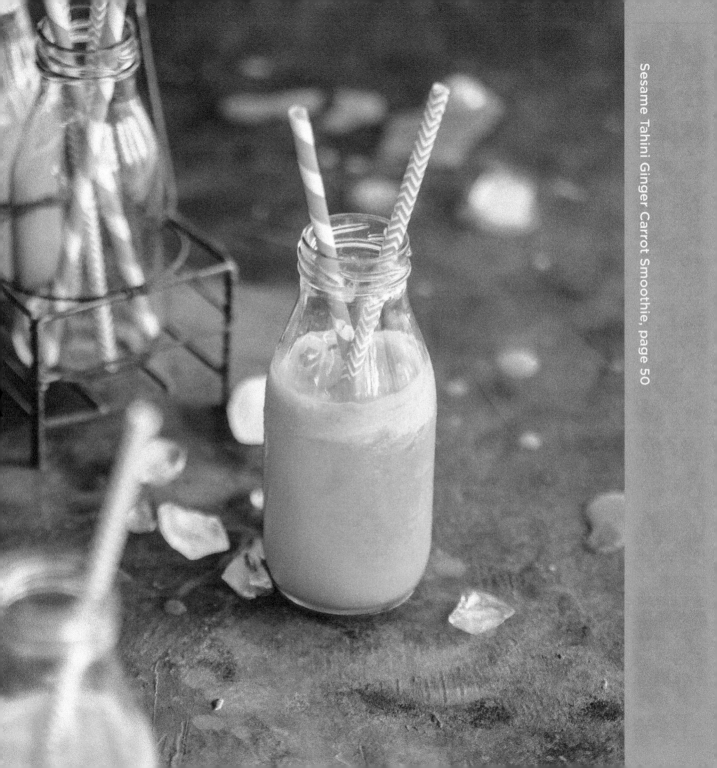

Cool Cucumber Yogurt Mint Smoothie, page 31

CHAPTER 2

HYDRATING AND RESTORATIVE

Keto flu got you feeling a little blah? This chapter has a variety of solutions to restore crucial electrolytes, quickly boost energy, and hydrate, hydrate, hydrate! Whether you've got a pounding headache or are feeling a little run-down, these recipes will help put the pep back in your step. To boost hydration and balance electrolytes, many of these smoothies are ice cube–based with electrolyte-rich ingredients like broth, chia seeds, citrus, cucumbers, and salt that do double duty by heightening the flavor. Other recipes in this section focus on restorative ingredients to support energy levels and overall health and wellness.

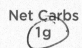
Almond and Chocolate Electrolyte Smoothie Booster Cubes

Prep time: 10 minutes, plus 6 hours to freeze | **Yield:** 8 servings | Super Low Carb

Smoothie cubes are a great way to boost the nutrition in your smoothies, and it's easy to tailor them to your needs. The electrolyte-dense ingredients in this recipe help keep you hydrated to make fighting keto flu a breeze. (The Ketorade Electrolyte Smoothie on page 23 can be frozen into smoothie cubes for the same purpose.)

2 cups unsweetened almond milk (or preferred dairy-free milk)

¼ cup unsweetened almond butter

3 tablespoons unsweetened cocoa powder

½ teaspoon sea salt

½ teaspoon potassium chloride salt alternative, such as Morton Lite Salt, NoSalt, or Nu Salt

1. In a blender, combine the almond milk, almond butter, cocoa powder, sea salt, and salt alternative.

2. Secure the lid and process at low speed until the ingredients are well combined, 1 to 2 minutes. If unblended ingredients remain or stick to the sides, use a spatula to scrape them down into the blended mixture and continue processing until thoroughly incorporated. The mixture will be a thin liquid.

3. Place an ice cube tray with 16 (1-ounce) wells on a flat surface. Fill each well to the top with the blended mixture. Transfer the tray to the freezer for a minimum of 5 to 6 hours.

4. To use, pop the frozen cubes out of the tray and add to the blender when mixing smoothies. For best results, add booster cubes as a final processing step (with or without ice), and process on the ice crush setting (or high speed).

Variation Tip: For even more magnesium, swap out the almond butter for pumpkin seed butter. For a protein boost, add a scoop of whey protein isolate powder.

Per Serving (2 cubes): Macronutrients: 71% Fat, 12% Protein, 17% Carbs; Calories: 62; Total Fat: 5g; Protein: 2g; Total Carbs: 3g; Fiber: 1g; Net Carbs: 1g

High-Fat Energy-Boosting Smoothie Cubes

Prep time: 10 minutes, plus 6 hours to freeze | **Yield:** 8 servings | Super Low Carb

Are you a meal prepper? Smoothie booster cubes are perfect for those who love to prep ingredients ahead of time for convenient use later. Like their name implies, these cubes are made for tossing into smoothie recipes to boost the energy content. You can also store them in your smoothie packs (see page 13).

1 (13.5-ounce) can unsweetened full-fat
   coconut milk

2 tablespoons MCT oil

½ teaspoon sea salt

1. In a blender, combine the coconut milk, MCT oil, and sea salt.

2. Secure the lid and process at low speed until the ingredients are fully incorporated, 1 to 2 minutes. If unblended ingredients remain or stick to the sides, use a spatula to scrape them down into the blended mixture and continue processing until thoroughly incorporated. The mixture will be a smooth, thick liquid.

3. Place an ice cube tray with 16 (1-ounce) wells on a flat surface. Fill each well to the top with the blended mixture. Transfer the tray to the freezer for a minimum of 5 to 6 hours.

4. To use, pop the frozen cubes out of the tray and add to the blender when mixing smoothies. For best results, add booster cubes as a final processing step (with or without ice), and process on the ice crush setting (or high speed).

Per Serving (2 cubes): Macronutrients: 95% Fat, 3% Protein, 2% Carbs; Calories: 114; Total Fat: 12g; Protein: 1g; Total Carbs: 2g; Fiber: 0g; Net Carbs: 2g

Bone Broth Smoothie

Prep time: 5 minutes | **Yield:** 1 serving | Super Low Carb

Bone broth is known for its nourishing, therapeutic properties and can be enjoyed as part of a ketogenic diet to support hydration and electrolyte balance. In fact, many keto folks love their broth, so I had to include this recipe! This savory collagen-rich smoothie is a feel-good elixir you'll want to make again and again.

1 cup beef or chicken bone broth, chilled

Juice of ½ lemon

2 tablespoons collagen hydroly-sate powder

⅛ teaspoon sea salt

2 tablespoons ghee, melted and slightly cooled

1 cup crushed or cubed ice

1. In a blender, combine the bone broth, lemon juice, collagen powder, and sea salt.

2. Secure the lid and process at high speed until the ingredients are well combined, about 1 minute.

3. While the blender is running, slowly pour in the melted ghee through the opening in the lid to prevent clumping. If unblended ingredients remain or stick to the sides, use a spatula to scrape them down into the blended mixture and continue processing until thoroughly incorporated. The mixture will be a thin, frothy liquid.

4. Add the ice to the blender, close the lid, and process on the ice crush setting (or high speed) until the ingredients are smooth and the ice is thoroughly incorporated, 1 to 2 minutes. The smoothie should have a thick, viscous consistency.

5. Serve immediately.

Variation Tip: If you don't have bone broth, use your favorite stock or broth instead. You can also enjoy this beverage warm—skip the ice and heat over the stovetop instead of whipping it up in the blender.

Per Serving: Macronutrients: 76% Fat, 21% Protein, 3% Carbs; Calories: 302; Total Fat: 26g; Protein: 18g; Total Carbs: 3g; Fiber: 0g; Net Carbs: 3g

Creamy Chai Tea Smoothie

Prep time: 5 minutes | **Yield:** 1 serving | High Fat, Super Low Carb

Chai tea contains many spices that provide a wide range of health benefits, including blood sugar management, reduced inflammation, and antioxidant protection. However, traditional chai tea is not keto-friendly due to the high quantities of milk and sugar in the beverage. This smoothie captures the essence of chai tea flavors without loading up on carbs.

1 cup black tea, brewed and cooled

¼ cup heavy (whipping) cream

1 tablespoon MCT oil

½ teaspoon vanilla extract

¼ teaspoon ground cinnamon

¼ teaspoon ground cardamom

⅛ teaspoon ground nutmeg

⅛ teaspoon ground cloves

1 cup crushed or cubed ice

1. In a blender, combine the black tea, heavy cream, MCT oil, vanilla, cinnamon, cardamom, nutmeg, and cloves.

2. Secure the lid and process at high speed until the ingredients are smooth and well combined, 1 to 2 minutes. If unblended ingredients remain or stick to the sides, use a spatula to scrape them down into the blended mixture and continue processing until thoroughly incorporated. The mixture will be a thin liquid.

3. Add the ice to the blender, close the lid, and process on the ice crush setting (or high speed) until the ingredients are smooth and the ice is thoroughly incorporated, 1 to 2 minutes. The smoothie should have a thick, creamy consistency.

4. Serve immediately.

Variation Tip: Black teas are most popularly used in chai teas, but feel free to experiment with this recipe—green tea, oolong, rooibos, yerba mate, or other herbal teas can stand in for the black tea.

Per Serving: Macronutrients: 94% Fat, 2% Protein, 4% Carbs; Calories: 346; Total Fat: 36g; Protein: 2g; Total Carbs: 4g; Fiber: 1g; Net Carbs: 3g

Ketorade Electrolyte Smoothie

Prep time: 5 minutes | **Yield:** 1 serving | Super Low Carb

People often turn to sports drinks to rehydrate and replenish electrolytes, but they're usually filled with sugar to help athletes refuel quickly. Skip the sugary sports drinks and whip up your own ketorade. This smoothie delivers similar amounts of sodium and potassium as a sports drink while helping you rapidly refuel with fat instead of carbs.

1 cup cold water

Juice of ½ lemon

Juice of ½ lime

1½ tablespoons MCT oil

½ teaspoon monkfruit erythritol blend sweetener or preferred sweetener (optional)

⅛ teaspoon sea salt

⅛ teaspoon potassium chloride salt alternative, such as Morton Lite Salt, NoSalt, or Nu Salt

1 cup crushed or cubed ice

1. In a blender, combine the water, lemon juice, lime juice, MCT oil, sweetener (if desired), sea salt, and salt alternative.

2. Secure the lid and process at low speed until the ingredients are smooth and well combined, about 1 minute. If unblended ingredients remain or stick to the sides, use a spatula to scrape them down into the blended mixture and continue processing until thoroughly incorporated. The mixture will be a watery liquid.

3. Add the ice to the blender, close the lid, and process on the ice crush setting (or high speed) until the ingredients are smooth and the ice is thoroughly incorporated, about 2 minutes. The smoothie should have a slushy consistency.

4. Serve immediately.

Variation Tip: Consider adding a powdered magnesium supplement to the smoothie to increase potassium absorption and support electrolyte balance. Check the manufacturer's label for individual dosage instructions.

Per Serving: Macronutrients: 100% Fat, <1% Protein, <1% Carbs; Calories: 185; Total Fat: 21g; Protein: <1g; Total Carbs: 4g; Fiber: <1g; Net Carbs: 3g; Erythritol: 2g _dinner snack_

Red Raspberry Rooibos Tea Refresher

Prep time: 5 minutes | **Yield:** 1 serving | Super Low Carb

No matter how many different teas I try, I always come back to rooibos. It's earthy and light, with a natural sweetness that pairs well with other ingredients, making it an excellent smoothie base. It's full of antioxidants and other health-promoting compounds. Plus it's caffeine-free—enjoy as much as you'd like without getting the jitters!

1 cup rooibos tea, brewed and cooled

2 tablespoons MCT oil

½ cup fresh or frozen raspberries

1 cup crushed or cubed ice

1. In a blender, combine the rooibos tea, MCT oil, and raspberries.

2. Secure the lid and process at high speed until the ingredients are smooth and well combined, 1 to 2 minutes. If unblended ingredients remain or stick to the sides, use a spatula to scrape them down into the blended mixture and continue processing until thoroughly incorporated. The mixture will be a thin, slushy liquid.

3. Add the ice to the blender, close the lid, and process on the ice crush setting (or high speed) until the ingredients are smooth and the ice is thoroughly incorporated, 1 to 2 minutes. The smoothie should have a thick, slushy consistency.

4. Serve immediately.

Variation Tip: Add 2 tablespoons of heavy cream to add a rich, creamy texture and boost the energy content.

Per Serving: Macronutrients: 89% Fat, 1% Protein, 10% Carbs; Calories: 264; Total Fat: 28g; Protein: 1g; Total Carbs: 7g; Fiber: 4g; Net Carbs: 3g

Chia Fresca Smoothie

Prep time: 5 minutes | **Yield:** 1 serving | High Fat, Super Low Carb

Chia fresca originates from Mexico and Central America but has become a popular drink worldwide thanks largely to the book *Born to Run*, in which Indigenous endurance runners use the beverage for long-lasting hydration and energy. I've added a few extra ingredients to make this a keto-friendly smoothie. Feel free to adjust the sweetener as desired.

1 cup cold water

Juice of 1 lime

½ teaspoon monkfruit erythritol blend sweetener (or preferred sweetener)

Pinch Himalayan pink salt

1 tablespoon chia seeds

2 tablespoons coconut oil, melted and slightly cooled

1 cup crushed or cubed ice

1. In a blender, combine the water, lime juice, sweetener, pink salt, and chia seeds.

2. Secure the lid and process at high speed until the ingredients are well combined, about 2 minutes.

3. While the blender is running, slowly pour in the melted coconut oil through the opening in the lid to prevent clumping. The texture will become thicker and begin to gel as the chia seeds absorb the liquid. If unblended ingredients remain or stick to the sides, use a spatula to scrape them down into the blended mixture and continue processing until smooth.

4. Add the ice to the blender, close the lid, and process on the ice crush setting (or high speed) until the ingredients are smooth and the ice is thoroughly incorporated, about 2 minutes. The smoothie should have a thick, seedy, viscous consistency.

5. Serve immediately.

Variation Tip: Swap out the lime juice for a few tablespoons of a different citrus juice, like grapefruit or lemon.

Per Serving: Macronutrients: 89% Fat, 3% Protein, 8% Carbs; Calories: 302; Total Fat: 30g; Protein: 2g; Total Carbs: 10g; Fiber: 4g; Net Carbs: 4g; Erythritol: 2g

Blended Iced Matcha Green Tea Latte

Prep time: 5 minutes | **Yield:** 1 serving | High Fat, Super Low Carb

Have you ever had green tea ice cream? Smooth and creamy, it has a rich herbal flavor and a gentle sweetness. I love it so much. This smoothie reminds me of those qualities. The matcha powder benefits the flavor as well as the nutrition, thanks to so many antioxidants!

¾ **cup cold water**

¼ **cup heavy (whipping) cream**

1 **tablespoon MCT oil**

¼ **teaspoon vanilla extract**

2 **teaspoons matcha powder (green tea powder)**

½ **teaspoon monkfruit erythritol blend sweetener (optional)**

Pinch sea salt

1 **cup crushed or cubed ice**

1. In a blender, combine the water, heavy cream, MCT oil, vanilla, matcha powder, sweetener (if desired), and sea salt.

2. Secure the lid and process at high speed until the ingredients are smooth and well combined, 1 to 2 minutes. If unblended ingredients remain or stick to the sides, use a spatula to scrape them down into the blended mixture and continue processing until thoroughly incorporated. The mixture will be a thin liquid.

3. Add the ice to the blender, close the lid, and process on the ice crush setting (or high speed) until the ingredients are smooth and the ice is thoroughly incorporated, 1 to 2 minutes. The smoothie should have a thick, creamy consistency.

4. Serve immediately.

Variation Tip: Heavy cream can be replaced with your keto-friendly dairy-free milk of choice. I love pairing unsweetened almond milk with matcha tea.

Per Serving: Macronutrients: 95% Fat, 2% Protein, 3% Carbs; Calories: 342; Total Fat: 36g; Protein: 2g; Total Carbs: 6g; Fiber: 0g; Net Carbs: 4g; Erythritol: 2g

Lemon Mint Tomato Smoothie

Prep time: 5 minutes | **Yield:** 1 serving | Super Low Carb

Sugary fruits dominate the smoothie world, but I much prefer unexpected savory options, like tomatoes. Loaded with water, antioxidants, vitamins, and minerals, tomatoes improve nutrient density and hydration while keeping carbs in check.

1 cup cold water

Juice of ½ lemon

2 tablespoons avocado oil

2 tablespoons collagen hydrolysate powder

Pinch sea salt

2 tablespoons fresh mint leaves

1 medium tomato, quartered

1 cup crushed or cubed ice

1. In a blender, combine the water, lemon juice, avocado oil, collagen powder, sea salt, mint leaves, and tomato.

2. Secure the lid and process at low speed until the ingredients are smooth and well combined, 1 to 2 minutes. If unblended ingredients remain or stick to the sides, use a spatula to scrape them down into the blended mixture and continue processing until thoroughly incorporated. The mixture will be a thin liquid.

3. Add the ice to the blender, close the lid, and process on the ice crush setting (or high speed) until the ingredients are smooth and the ice is thoroughly incorporated, about 2 minutes. The smoothie should have a thick, slushy consistency.

4. Serve immediately.

Per Serving: Macronutrients: 80% Fat, 16% Protein, 4% Carbs; Calories: 316; Total Fat: 28g; Protein: 13g; Total Carbs: 7g; Fiber: 2g; Net Carbs: 5g

Spinach Turmeric Protein Smoothie

Prep time: 5 minutes | **Yield:** 1 serving | High Protein, Super Low Carb

This savory smoothie is one of my favorite health boosters. Rich in protein and electrolytes, it also contains potent compounds that support wellness and fight disease. For example, curcumin, the active compound in turmeric, can reduce inflammation and oxidative stress. Don't forget the black pepper—it contains piperine, which improves the absorption of curcumin.

1 cup cold water

Juice of ½ lemon

2 tablespoons extra-virgin olive oil

1 scoop whey protein isolate powder, unflavored

1 teaspoon ground turmeric (or 1 tablespoon grated fresh)

Pinch freshly ground black pepper

1 cup fresh spinach

1 cup crushed or cubed ice

1. In a blender, combine the water, lemon juice, olive oil, protein powder, turmeric, black pepper, and spinach.

2. Secure the lid and process at high speed until the ingredients are smooth and well combined, about 2 minutes. If unblended ingredients remain or stick to the sides, use a spatula to scrape them down into the blended mixture and continue processing until thoroughly incorporated. The mixture will be a thin liquid.

3. Add the ice to the blender, close the lid, and process on the ice crush setting (or high speed) until the ingredients are smooth and the ice is thoroughly incorporated, 1 to 2 minutes. The smoothie should have a thick, slushy consistency.

4. Serve immediately.

Per Serving: Macronutrients: 67% Fat, 27% Protein, 6% Carbs; Calories: 390; Total Fat: 29g; Protein: 26g; Total Carbs: 7g; Fiber: 2g; Net Carbs: 5g

Strawberry Lemonade Smoothie

Prep time: 5 minutes | **Yield:** 1 serving | Super Low Carb

This refreshing smoothie uses freshly squeezed lemon juice and frozen strawberries to achieve the iconic strawberry lemonade flavors. The fruit also provides an electrolyte boost from potassium, magnesium, and calcium. Keto-friendly sweetener balances the tart lemon without adding any sugar—feel free to adjust the sweetener as desired.

1 cup cold water

Juice of 1 lemon

2 tablespoons MCT oil

½ teaspoon monkfruit erythritol sweetener
  blend or preferred sweetener

⅛ teaspoon Himalayan pink salt

3 large frozen strawberries

1 cup crushed or cubed ice

1. In a blender, combine the water, lemon juice, MCT oil, sweetener, pink salt, and strawberries.

2. Secure the lid and process at high speed until the ingredients are smooth and well combined, about 2 minutes. If unblended ingredients remain or stick to the sides, use a spatula to scrape them down into the blended mixture and continue processing until thoroughly incorporated. The mixture will be a thin liquid.

3. Add the ice to the blender, close the lid, and process on the ice crush setting (or high speed) until the ingredients are smooth and the ice is thoroughly incorporated, about 2 minutes. The smoothie should have a thick, slushy consistency.

4. Serve immediately.

Variation Tip: If you prefer a lighter drink, skip the oil. If you don't have MCT oil on hand, avocado oil is a good neutral-flavored substitute.

Per Serving: Macronutrients: 97% Fat, 1% Protein, 2% Carbs; Calories: 261; Total Fat: 28g; Protein: 1g; Total Carbs: 9g; Fiber: 1g; Net Carbs: 6g; Erythritol: 2g

Superfood Spirulina Smoothie

Prep time: 5 minutes | **Yield:** 1 serving | High Fat, High Protein, Super Low Carb

I always try to maximize nutrient density in my smoothies. An easy way to accomplish this is by using "superfoods," which are foods and dietary supplements packed with nutritional value, like dark leafy greens, avocado, berries, nuts, seeds, and nutritional powders.

1 cup cold water

Juice of ½ lemon

1 tablespoon MCT oil or extra-virgin olive oil

2 tablespoons spirulina powder

2 tablespoons collagen hydrolysate powder

2 tablespoons chia seeds

½ avocado, peeled, pitted, and cut into chunks

1 cup crushed or cubed ice

1. In a blender, combine the water, lemon juice, oil, spirulina powder, collagen powder, chia seeds, and avocado.

2. Secure the lid and process at high speed until the ingredients are smooth and well combined, about 2 minutes. The mixture will thicken and begin to gel as the chia seeds absorb the liquid. If unblended ingredients remain or stick to the sides, use a spatula to scrape them down into the blended mixture and continue processing until thoroughly incorporated. The mixture will be a viscous liquid.

3. Add the ice to the blender, close the lid, and process on the ice crush setting (or high speed) until the ingredients are smooth and the ice is thoroughly incorporated, 1 to 2 minutes. The smoothie should have a gelled, slushy consistency.

4. Serve immediately.

Variation Tip: Not a fan of spirulina? No problem! Other nutritional powders like chlorella, matcha, or moringa make a great superfood swap with a subtler flavor.

Per Serving: Macronutrients: 69% Fat, 21% Protein, 10% Carbs; Calories: 405; Total Fat: 31g; Protein: 21g; Total Carbs: 18g; Fiber: 12g; Net Carbs: 6g

Cool Cucumber Yogurt Mint Smoothie

Prep time: 5 minutes | **Yield:** 1 serving | Super Low Carb

Cucumber and mint is one of my favorite flavor combinations—add a little yogurt, and there's nothing more refreshing! Let this creamy smoothie cool you off while you load up on potassium, magnesium, and calcium. I don't peel the cucumber, but you can if you want a more consistent texture.

1 cup cold water

2 tablespoons plain full-fat Greek yogurt

2 tablespoons MCT oil

¼ teaspoon mint extract (optional)

¼ cup fresh mint leaves

1 medium cucumber, cut into large chunks

1 cup crushed or cubed ice

1. In a blender, combine the water, yogurt, MCT oil, mint extract (if desired), mint leaves, and cucumber.

2. Secure the lid and process at high speed until the ingredients are smooth and well combined, 1 to 2 minutes. If unblended ingredients remain or stick to the sides, use a spatula to scrape them down into the blended mixture and continue processing until thoroughly incorporated. The mixture will be like a thin yogurt sauce.

3. Add the ice to the blender, close the lid, and process on the ice crush setting (or high speed) until the ingredients are smooth and the ice is thoroughly incorporated, about 2 minutes. The smoothie should have a thick, creamy consistency.

4. Serve immediately.

Per Serving: Macronutrients: 91% Fat, 5% Protein, 4% Carbs; Calories: 295; Total Fat: 30g; Protein: 4g; Total Carbs: 10g; Fiber: 3g; Net Carbs: 7g

Cucumber Agua Fresca Smoothie

Prep time: 5 minutes | **Yield:** 1 serving | Super Low Carb

Agua fresca is a blended fruit juice typically strained and mixed with sugar, honey, or maple syrup. It's hydrating, refreshing, and full of electrolytes; it's also super high in carbs. Here, we're using keto ingredients and skipping the strainer to retain all the healthy fiber and nutrients. Feel free to adjust the sweetener as desired.

1 cup cold water

Juice of ½ lime

2 tablespoons avocado oil

½ teaspoon maple extract (optional)

½ teaspoon monkfruit erythritol sweetener (or sweetener of choice)

1 medium cucumber, cut into large chunks

1 cup crushed or cubed ice

1. In a blender, combine the water, lime juice, avocado oil, maple extract (if desired), sweetener, and cucumber.

2. Secure the lid and process at high speed until the ingredients are smooth and well combined, 1 to 2 minutes. If unblended ingredients remain or stick to the sides, use a spatula to scrape them down into the blended mixture and continue processing until thoroughly incorporated. The mixture will be a thick liquid.

3. Add the ice to the blender, close the lid, and process on the ice crush setting (or high speed) until the ingredients are smooth and the ice is thoroughly incorporated, about 2 minutes. The smoothie should have a thick, slushy consistency.

4. Serve immediately.

Variation Tip: Agua fresca is traditionally made with a variety of fruits. Try swapping the cucumber with blackberries, strawberries, raspberries, blueberries, or avocado to add variation while keeping it keto-friendly.

Per Serving: Macronutrients: 90% Fat, 3% Protein, 7% Carbs; Calories: 280; Total Fat: 28g; Protein: 2g; Total Carbs: 12g; Fiber: 3g; Net Carbs: 7g; Erythritol: 2g

Dill Pickle Smoothie

Prep time: 5 minutes | **Yield:** 1 serving | High Protein

Pickles may chase away more headaches than aspirin in the keto community. Their high sodium content makes pickles a popular remedy for the keto flu. Some people even sip pickle juice straight from the container! The Greek yogurt in this smoothie curbs the salty flavor while upgrading the electrolyte content.

1 cup plain full-fat Greek yogurt

¼ cup unsweetened dill pickle brine

1 tablespoon extra-virgin olive oil

1 tablespoon chopped fresh dill weed

1 large dill pickle, cut into chunks

1 cup crushed or cubed ice

1. In a blender, combine the yogurt, pickle brine, olive oil, dill weed, and pickle.

2. Secure the lid and process at low speed until the ingredients are smooth and well combined, 1 to 2 minutes. If unblended ingredients remain or stick to the sides, use a spatula to scrape them down into the blended mixture and continue processing until thoroughly incorporated. The mixture will be like a thick yogurt sauce.

3. Add the ice to the blender, close the lid, and process on the ice crush setting (or high speed) until the ingredients are smooth and the ice is thoroughly incorporated, about 2 minutes. The smoothie should have a thick, creamy consistency, similar to a soft-serve shake.

4. Serve immediately.

Variation Tip: Swap the Greek yogurt out for cold water and increase the brine. This will make a pickle juice slush, similar to the one served at the Sonic restaurant chain.

Per Serving: Macronutrients: 64% Fat, 24% Protein, 12% Carbs; Calories: 351; Total Fat: 25g; Protein: 21g; Total Carbs: 12g; Fiber: 1g; Net Carbs: 11g

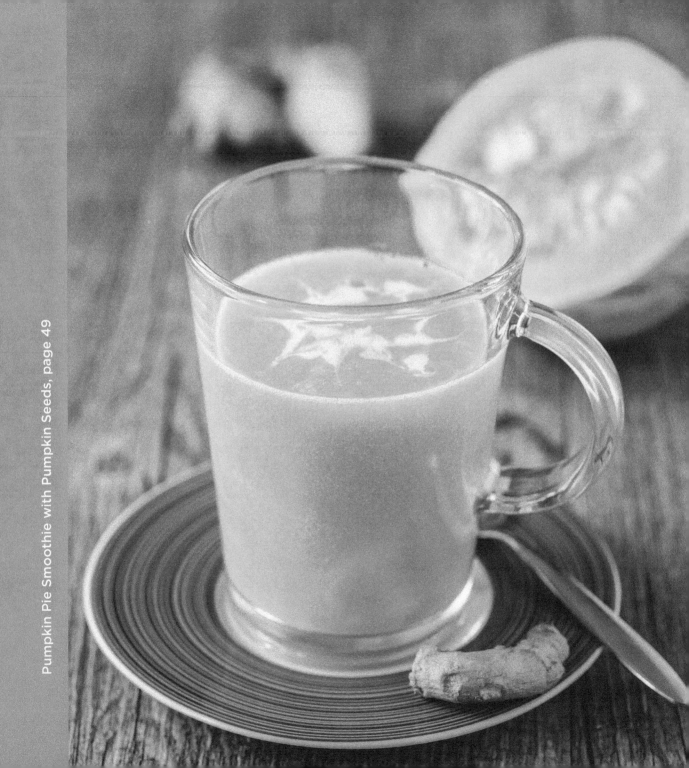

Pumpkin Pie Smoothie with Pumpkin Seeds, page 49

CHAPTER 3

NUTTY (NUTS AND SEEDS)

Nuts and seeds are an excellent way to boost the nutrition content of your smoothies with healthy fats, fiber, protein, and a plethora of micronutrients, including magnesium, potassium, iron, zinc, selenium, and vitamins E and B. They are easy to incorporate into smoothies of all kinds, from sweet to savory. Nut and seed milks serve as a liquid base in many of the smoothies featured in this chapter; however, blended butters, whole nuts, and seeds are also prominent ingredients in the recipes. If you enjoy the earthy flavors of nuts and seeds—such as almonds, macadamia, pecans, walnuts, chia, hemp, pumpkin, and sunflower—this chapter is for you.

Nutty Horchata Smoothie

Prep time: 5 minutes | **Yield:** 1 serving | High Fat, Super Low Carb

Horchata, or orxata, is a sweetened plant-based milk beverage bursting with vanilla and cinnamon flavor. In Mexico and the Americas, it's traditionally made with rice milk, but the Spanish version uses a nutty base. Macadamia milk and keto-friendly sweetener make this horchata low-carb—just blend with ice for a frozen smoothie treat.

1 cup unsweetened macadamia nut milk (or preferred dairy-free milk)

⅓ cup heavy (whipping) cream

1 teaspoon vanilla extract

½ teaspoon monkfruit erythritol blend sweetener (or preferred sweetener)

½ teaspoon ground cinnamon

1 cup crushed or cubed ice

1 cinnamon stick, for garnish (optional)

1. In a blender, combine the milk, heavy cream, vanilla, sweetener, and cinnamon.

2. Secure the lid and process at high speed until the ingredients are smooth and well combined, 1 to 2 minutes. If unblended ingredients remain or stick to the sides, use a spatula to scrape them down into the blended mixture and continue processing until thoroughly incorporated. The mixture will be a thin liquid.

3. Add the ice to the blender, close the lid, and process on the ice crush setting (or high speed) until the ingredients are smooth and the ice is thoroughly incorporated, 1 to 2 minutes. The smoothie should have a thick, creamy consistency.

4. Pour the mixture into a serving glass, garnish with the cinnamon stick (if desired), and enjoy immediately.

Variation Tip: Make this smoothie nut-free by swapping the macadamia nut milk with coconut milk beverage.

Per Serving: Macronutrients: 98% Fat, 1% Protein, 1% Carbs; Calories: 336; Total Fat: 37g; Protein: 3g; Total Carbs: 7g; Fiber: 2g; Net Carbs: 3g; Erythritol: 2g

Butter Pecan Smoothie

Prep time: 5 minutes | **Yield:** 1 serving | High Fat, Super Low Carb

Do you ever want to eat a big bowl of ice cream but don't because it's a sugar bomb? If you can relate, this butter pecan smoothie will really hit the spot. It's rich and creamy, just like your favorite frozen treat, with a fraction of the carbs.

1 cup unsweetened walnut milk (or preferred dairy-free milk)

2 tablespoons heavy (whipping) cream

1 teaspoon vanilla extract

½ teaspoon monkfruit erythritol blend
sweetener (or preferred sweetener)

⅓ cup pecans, chopped

1 tablespoon butter or ghee, melted and
slightly cooled

1 cup crushed or cubed ice

1. In a blender, combine the walnut milk, heavy cream, vanilla, sweetener, and pecans.

2. Secure the lid and process at high speed until the ingredients are well combined, 1 to 2 minutes.

3. While the blender is running, slowly pour in the melted butter through the opening in the lid to prevent clumping. If unblended ingredients remain or stick to the sides, use a spatula to scrape them down into the blended mixture and continue processing until thoroughly incorporated. The mixture will be a thick liquid.

4. Add the ice to the blender, close the lid, and process on the ice crush setting (or high speed) until the ingredients are smooth and the ice is thoroughly incorporated into the mixture, 1 to 2 minutes. The smoothie should have a thick, creamy consistency with tiny pieces of pecan distributed throughout.

5. Serve immediately.

Per Serving: Macronutrients: 90% Fat, 5% Protein, 5% Carbs; Calories: 587; Total Fat: 59g; Protein: 7g; Total Carbs: 9g; Fiber: 4g; Net Carbs: 4g; Erythritol: 2g

Almond Butter and Shredded Coconut Smoothie

Prep time: 5 minutes | **Yield:** 1 serving | Super Low Carb

The natural sweetness of coconut paired with woody, earthy almonds makes for a fantastic smoothie to start your day. The subtle sweetness from the natural ingredients is enhanced with a pinch of sea salt to provide the perfect balance of sweet and salty flavors.

1½ cups unsweetened coconut milk beverage

2 tablespoons almond butter

½ teaspoon vanilla extract

Pinch sea salt

2 tablespoons unsweetened dried coconut flakes

1 cup crushed or cubed ice (optional)

1. In a blender, combine the coconut milk beverage, almond butter, vanilla, sea salt, and coconut flakes.

2. Secure the lid and process at high speed until the ingredients are smooth and well combined, 1 to 2 minutes. If unblended ingredients remain or stick to the sides, use a spatula to scrape them down into the blended mixture and continue processing until thoroughly incorporated. The mixture will be a thick liquid.

3. If desired, add the ice to the blender, close the lid, and process on the ice crush setting (or high speed) until the ingredients are smooth and the ice is thoroughly incorporated, 1 to 2 minutes. The smoothie should have a thick consistency.

4. Serve immediately.

Per Serving: Macronutrients: 82% Fat, 11% Protein, 7% Carbs; Calories: 339; Total Fat: 31g; Protein: 9g; Total Carbs: 10g; Fiber: 5g; Net Carbs: 5g

Chocolate Hazelnut Smoothie

Prep time: 5 minutes | **Yield:** 1 serving | High Fat, Super Low Carb

Nutella lovers rejoice! This smoothie packs the sweet hazelnut-cocoa flavors of the famous spread in a keto-friendly package—delicious nutty goodness without any of the added sugars.

1 cup unsweetened hazelnut milk (or preferred dairy-free milk)

1 tablespoon avocado oil

1 tablespoon unsweetened cocoa powder

½ teaspoon monkfruit erythritol blend sweetener (or preferred sweetener)

Pinch sea salt

⅓ cup hazelnuts

1 cup crushed or cubed ice (optional)

1. In a blender, combine the hazelnut milk, avocado oil, cocoa powder, sweetener, sea salt, and hazelnuts.

2. Secure the lid and process at high speed until the ingredients are smooth and well combined, 1 to 2 minutes. If unblended ingredients remain or stick to the sides, use a spatula to scrape them down into the blended mixture and continue processing until thoroughly incorporated. The mixture will be a thick liquid.

3. If desired, add the ice to the blender, close the lid, and process on the ice crush setting (or high speed) until the ingredients are smooth and the ice is thoroughly incorporated, 1 to 2 minutes. The smoothie should have a thick consistency.

4. Serve immediately.

Per Serving: Macronutrients: 89% Fat, 8% Protein, 3% Carbs; Calories: 513; Total Fat: 50g; Protein: 11g; Total Carbs: 14g; Fiber: 6g; Net Carbs: 6g; Erythritol: 2g

Mint Macadamia Nut and Coconut Cream Smoothie

Prep time: 5 minutes | **Yield:** 1 serving | High Fat, Super Low Carb

Creamy coconut and buttery macadamia boost the fat content of this smoothie while providing a rich, decadent base. Fresh mint leaves brighten the flavor and add a cooling effect.

½ **cup unsweetened macadamia nut milk (or coconut milk beverage)**

½ **cup unsweetened coconut cream**

⅓ **cup macadamia nuts**

1 **teaspoon fresh mint leaves (or** ½ **teaspoon mint extract)**

1 **cup crushed or cubed ice (optional)**

1. In a blender, combine the macadamia nut milk, coconut cream, macadamia nuts, and mint leaves.

2. Secure the lid and process at high speed until the ingredients are smooth and well combined, 1 to 2 minutes. If unblended ingredients remain or stick to the sides, use a spatula to scrape them down into the blended mixture and continue processing until thoroughly incorporated. The mixture will be a thick, creamy liquid.

3. If desired, add the ice to the blender, close the lid, and process on the ice crush setting (or high speed) until the ingredients are smooth and the ice is thoroughly incorporated, 1 to 2 minutes. The smoothie should have a thick, creamy consistency.

4. Serve immediately.

Per Serving: Macronutrients: 93% Fat, 3% Protein, 4% Carbs; Calories: 583; Total Fat: 60g; Protein: 4g; Total Carbs: 9g; Fiber: 4g; Net Carbs: 6g

Spicy Hazelnut and Almond Milk Smoothie

Prep time: 5 minutes | **Yield:** 1 serving | Super Low Carb

Adding a little heat to your smoothies is an excellent way to kick the flavor up a notch and give your health and metabolism a little boost. Capsaicin, the active component of chile peppers, can help you burn more energy, reduce hunger, aid digestion, and combat inflammation.

1 cup unsweetened almond milk (or preferred dairy-free milk)

½ teaspoon vanilla extract

½ teaspoon monkfruit erythritol blend sweetener (or preferred sweetener)

¼ teaspoon cayenne pepper

¼ teaspoon ground chipotle chili pepper (or preferred chili powder)

⅓ cup hazelnuts

1 cup crushed or cubed ice (optional)

1. In a blender, combine the almond milk, vanilla, sweetener, cayenne, chipotle, and hazelnuts.

2. Secure the lid and process at high speed until the ingredients are smooth and well combined, 1 to 2 minutes. If unblended ingredients remain or stick to the sides, use a spatula to scrape them down into the blended mixture and continue processing until thoroughly incorporated. The mixture will be a thick liquid.

3. If desired, add the ice to the blender, close the lid, and process on the ice crush setting (or high speed) until the ingredients are smooth and the ice is thoroughly incorporated, 1 to 2 minutes. The smoothie should have a thick consistency.

4. Serve immediately.

Variation Tip: Can't handle the heat? No worries! Omit the chili pepper and opt for other spices. Cinnamon, allspice, nutmeg, and cloves are great substitutes to tone this recipe down.

Per Serving: Macronutrients: 83% Fat, 10% Protein, 7% Carbs; Calories: 325; Total Fat: 30g; Protein: 8g; Total Carbs: 13g; Fiber: 5g; Net Carbs: 6g; Erythritol: 2g

No-Oats Oatmeal Smoothie

Prep time: 5 minutes | **Yield:** 1 serving | High Protein, Super Low Carb

Oatmeal is a popular way to kick-start a day and makes a fabulous smoothie addition, but oats are a no-go for keto. Luckily, we can use nuts and seeds to mimic the flavors and texture of oatmeal without racking up the carbs.

1 cup unsweetened almond milk (or preferred dairy-free milk)

2 tablespoons ground flaxseed

1 tablespoon almond flour

½ teaspoon ground cinnamon

2 tablespoons hemp hearts

2 tablespoons chia seeds

1 cup crushed or cubed ice (optional)

1. In a blender, combine the almond milk, flaxseed, almond flour, cinnamon, hemp hearts, and chia seeds.

2. Secure the lid and process at high speed until the ingredients are smooth and well combined, 1 to 2 minutes. If unblended ingredients remain or stick to the sides, use a spatula to scrape them down into the blended mixture and continue processing until thoroughly incorporated. The mixture will be a thick, seedy liquid.

3. If desired, add the ice to the blender, close the lid, and process on the ice crush setting (or high speed) until the ingredients are smooth and the ice is thoroughly incorporated, 1 to 2 minutes. The smoothie should have a thick consistency with small bits of seeds distributed throughout.

4. Serve immediately.

Variation Tip: This recipe makes a great "oatmeal" smoothie base that can be customized to your liking. Try adding sweetener and maple extract or strawberries and cream, or mix in peanut butter and sugar-free chocolate chips for variety!

Per Serving: Macronutrients: 66% Fat, 16% Protein, 18% Carbs; Calories: 367; Total Fat: 27g; Protein: 15g; Total Carbs: 19g; Fiber: 13g; Net Carbs: 6g

Pumpkin Seed and Hemp Heart Smoothie

Prep time: 5 minutes | **Yield:** 1 serving | High Protein, Super Low Carb

I love to sneak pumpkin seeds into my meals whenever I can. They are delicious and loaded with magnesium, an important electrolyte that can be hard to source from low-carb foods. The nutrient-dense hemp seed adds an earthy, nutty flavor and creamy consistency.

1 cup unsweetened hemp seed milk

1 teaspoon extra-virgin olive oil

2 tablespoons collagen hydrolysate powder

¼ teaspoon cayenne pepper

Pinch sea salt

¼ cup pumpkin seeds, unshelled

2 tablespoons hemp hearts

1 cup crushed or cubed ice (optional)

1. In a blender, combine the hemp milk, olive oil, collagen powder, cayenne, sea salt, pumpkin seeds, and hemp hearts.

2. Secure the lid and process at high speed until the ingredients are smooth and well combined, 1 to 2 minutes. If unblended ingredients remain or stick to the sides, use a spatula to scrape them down into the blended mixture and continue processing until thoroughly incorporated. The mixture will be a thick, seedy liquid.

3. If desired, add the ice to the blender, close the lid, and process on the ice crush setting (or high speed) until the ingredients are smooth and the ice is thoroughly incorporated. The smoothie should have a thick consistency with small bits of seeds distributed throughout.

4. Serve immediately.

Per Serving: Macronutrients: 66% Fat, 27% Protein, 7% Carbs; Calories: 356; Total Fat: 26g; Protein: 24g; Total Carbs: 11g; Fiber: 4g; Net Carbs: 7g

Pine Nut Cauliflower Smoothie

Prep time: 5 minutes | **Yield:** 1 serving | Super Low Carb

If you haven't tried cauliflower in a smoothie yet, you're in for a treat! I love to use it to boost the nutritional value and texture in place of ice cubes. Cauliflower's mild flavor is relatively neutral when blended with other ingredients, so it won't compete for the spotlight.

1 cup unsweetened coconut milk beverage

Juice of ½ lime

Pinch sea salt

¼ cup pine nuts

1 cup chopped or riced frozen cauliflower

1. In a blender, combine the coconut milk beverage, lime juice, sea salt, and pine nuts.

2. Secure the lid and process at high speed until the ingredients are smooth and well combined, 1 to 2 minutes. If unblended ingredients remain or stick to the sides, use a spatula to scrape them down into the blended mixture and continue processing until thoroughly incorporated. The mixture will be a thin liquid.

3. Add the frozen cauliflower to the blender, close the lid, and process on the ice crush setting (or high speed) until the ingredients are smooth and the cauliflower is thoroughly incorporated, 1 to 2 minutes. The smoothie should have a thick consistency with tiny pieces of pine nuts distributed throughout.

4. Serve immediately.

Variation Tip: If you don't have pine nuts on hand, almonds, macadamia nuts, hazelnuts, pecans, or walnuts would be a fantastic swap. If you want a nut-free recipe, consider using hemp, pumpkin, or sunflower seeds instead.

Per Serving: Macronutrients: 81% Fat, 10% Protein, 9% Carbs; Calories: 288; Total Fat: 26g; Protein: 7g; Total Carbs: 13g; Fiber: 6g; Net Carbs: 7g

Cinnamon Walnut Cranberry Smoothie

Prep time: 5 minutes | **Yield:** 1 serving | High Fat, Super Low Carb

Rich, earthy walnuts, tart cranberries, and sweet, woody cinnamon flavors come together in this autumn-inspired recipe. Fresh cranberries are harvested in the fall, and that's when they can be found in the grocery store, but feel free to use frozen ones year-round.

1 cup unsweetened walnut milk (or preferred dairy-free milk)

½ teaspoon ground cinnamon

½ cup fresh or frozen cranberries

⅓ cup walnut halves

1 cup crushed or cubed ice (optional)

1. In a blender, combine the walnut milk, cinnamon, cranberries, and walnuts.

2. Secure the lid and process at high speed until the ingredients are smooth and well combined, 1 to 2 minutes. If unblended ingredients remain or stick to the sides, use a spatula to scrape them down into the blended mixture and continue processing until thoroughly incorporated. The mixture will be a thin liquid.

3. If desired, add the ice to the blender, close the lid, and process on the ice crush setting (or high speed) until the ingredients are smooth and the ice is thoroughly incorporated, 1 to 2 minutes. The smoothie should have a thick consistency with tiny pieces of walnut distributed throughout.

4. Serve immediately.

Variation Tip: Add a splash of freshly squeezed orange juice to enhance and sweeten the tart cranberry flavor.

Per Serving: Macronutrients: 82% Fat, 9% Protein, 9% Carbs; Calories: 364; Total Fat: 33g; Protein: 8g; Total Carbs: 13g; Fiber: 5g; Net Carbs: 8g

The PB&J: Peanut Butter and "Jelly" Smoothie

Prep time: 5 minutes | **Yield:** 1 serving | High Protein, Super Low Carb

This protein-packed smoothie delivers the famous PB&J flavor combination of everyone's favorite sandwich—without all the carbs. Surprisingly filling, this recipe is loaded with nutrients and an extra protein boost, making it a satisfying meal replacement or ideal post-workout shake. You'll love this healthy take on the sugar-loaded classic.

1 cup unsweetened vanilla almond milk (or preferred dairy-free milk)

2 tablespoons natural peanut butter, divided

1 scoop unflavored whey protein isolate powder

2 large frozen strawberries

1. In a blender, combine the almond milk, 11/2 tablespoons of peanut butter, the protein powder, and strawberries.

2. Secure the lid and process at high speed until the ingredients are smooth and well combined, 1 to 2 minutes. If unblended ingredients remain or stick to the sides, use a spatula to scrape them down into the blended mixture and continue processing until thoroughly incorporated. The mixture will be a thin liquid.

3. Pour the mixture into a serving glass. Microwave the remaining ½ tablespoon of peanut butter in a microwave-safe dish on high until the peanut butter softens to a pourable liquid, about 30 seconds. Stir the warm peanut butter and drizzle it over the prepared smoothie.

4. Serve immediately.

Variation Tip: Fresh strawberries will work if you don't have frozen ones, but the resulting smoothie will be thinner. To thicken up the drink, add ¼ cup of ice to the blender before processing.

Per Serving: Macronutrients: 50% Fat, 41% Protein, 9% Carbs; Calories: 345; Total Fat: 19g; Protein: 35g; Total Carbs: 12g; Fiber: 3g; Net Carbs: 8g; Erythritol: 0.13g

Pecan Carrot Cake Shake

Prep time: 5 minutes | **Yield:** 1 serving | High Fat, Super Low Carb

This dessertlike smoothie plays up the flavors of carrot cake, complete with cheesecake frosting and pecan topping. Don't be fooled by the decadent flavor; this recipe is perfectly keto-friendly! It's low in carbs and high-fat and loaded with nutrients like vitamin A, potassium, manganese, zinc, magnesium, and fiber.

1 cup unsweetened walnut milk (or preferred dairy-free milk)

2 tablespoons cream cheese, softened

½ teaspoon monkfruit erythritol blend sweetener (or preferred sweetener)

½ teaspoon ground cinnamon

⅓ cup pecans

½ cup fresh or frozen carrots

1 cup crushed or cubed ice (optional)

1. In a blender, combine the walnut milk, cream cheese, sweetener, cinnamon, pecans, and carrots.

2. Secure the lid and process at high speed until the ingredients are smooth and well combined, 1 to 2 minutes. If unblended ingredients remain or stick to the sides, use a spatula to scrape them down into the blended mixture and continue processing until thoroughly incorporated. The mixture will be a thick, creamy liquid.

3. If desired, add the ice to the blender, close the lid, and process on the ice crush setting (or high speed) until the ingredients are smooth and the ice is thoroughly incorporated, 1 to 2 minutes. The smoothie should have a thick, creamy consistency with tiny pieces of pecan distributed throughout.

4. Serve immediately.

Per Serving: Macronutrients: 85% Fat, 7% Protein, 8% Carbs; Calories: 500; Total Fat: 47g; Protein: 9g; Total Carbs: 17g; Fiber: 6g; Net Carbs: 9g; Erythritol: 2g

Pumpkin Pie Smoothie with Pumpkin Seeds

Prep time: 5 minutes | **Yield:** 1 serving | High Fat, Super Low Carb

This smoothie embodies pumpkin spice season, when the kids are back in school, the leaves are falling from the trees in orange and red piles, and Halloween is just around the corner. Luckily, you don't have to wait until fall to enjoy this recipe—it's great year-round.

1 cup unsweetened almond milk (or preferred dairy-free milk)

1 tablespoon pumpkin seed oil (or preferred oil)

¼ cup canned pumpkin puree

½ teaspoon vanilla extract

½ teaspoon pumpkin pie spice

½ teaspoon monkfruit erythritol blend sweetener or preferred sweetener (optional)

¼ cup pumpkin seeds, shelled

1 cup crushed or cubed ice (optional)

1. In a blender, combine the almond milk, oil, pumpkin puree, vanilla, pumpkin pie spice, sweetener (if desired), and pumpkin seeds.

2. Secure the lid and process at high speed until the ingredients are smooth and well combined, 1 to 2 minutes. If unblended ingredients remain or stick to the sides, use a spatula to scrape them down into the blended mixture and continue processing until thoroughly incorporated. The mixture will be a thick liquid.

3. If desired, add the ice to the blender, close the lid, and process on the ice crush setting (or high speed) until the ingredients are smooth and the ice is thoroughly incorporated, 1 to 2 minutes. The smoothie should have a thick consistency with tiny pieces of pumpkin seeds distributed throughout.

4. Serve immediately.

Variation Tip: Add some fresh ginger for a warm bite.

Per Serving: Macronutrients: 77% Fat, 10% Protein, 13% Carbs; Calories: 351; Total Fat: 30g; Protein: 9g; Total Carbs: 15g; Fiber: 4g; Net Carbs: 9g; Erythritol: 2g

Sesame Tahini Ginger Carrot Smoothie

Prep time: 5 minutes | **Yield:** 1 serving | High Protein

Sesame seed milk provides a subtle nutty base for the earthy tahini, peppery ginger, and sweet carrot. Combined, the flavors lean toward bitter, which can be an enjoyable break from sweet and savory. If you find it overpowering, try adding sweetener.

1 cup unsweetened sesame seed milk (or preferred dairy-free milk)

2 tablespoons tahini

2 tablespoons collagen hydrolysate powder

1 teaspoon ground ginger

Pinch sea salt

½ cup fresh or frozen sliced carrots

1 cup crushed or cubed ice (optional)

1. In a blender, combine the sesame seed milk, tahini, collagen powder, ginger, sea salt, and carrots.

2. Secure the lid and process at high speed until the ingredients are smooth and well combined, 1 to 2 minutes. If unblended ingredients remain or stick to the sides, use a spatula to scrape them down into the blended mixture and continue processing until thoroughly incorporated. The mixture will be a thin liquid.

3. If desired, add the ice to the blender, close the lid, and process on the ice crush setting (or high speed) until the ingredients are smooth and the ice is thoroughly incorporated, 1 to 2 minutes. The smoothie should have a thick consistency.

4. Serve immediately.

Variation Tip: Add turmeric to the smoothie to boost health benefits and brighten the orange coloring. Don't forget to add a pinch of black pepper, too, for the full benefit (see page 28 for a note about curcumin and piperine). Hemp seed or almond milk is a good alternative if sesame seed milk is unavailable.

Per Serving: Macronutrients: 54% Fat, 24% Protein, 22% Carbs; Calories: 349; Total Fat: 21g; Protein: 26g; Total Carbs: 17g; Fiber: 6g; Net Carbs: 11g

The Health Nut

Prep time: 5 minutes | **Yield:** 1 serving | High Protein

Of all the smoothies in this book, this one has been in my regular rotation longest. *That's* because I always have the ingredients on hand, so it's ultra-convenient. I encourage you to find a few recipes you absolutely love and keep those ingredients stocked (see page 6 for pantry advice).

1 cup unsweetened almond milk (or preferred dairy-free milk)

2 tablespoons almond butter

½ teaspoon vanilla extract

1 scoop whey protein isolate powder
(or preferred protein powder)

¼ cup fresh or frozen blueberries

1 cup crushed or cubed
ice (optional)

1. In a blender, combine the almond milk, almond butter, vanilla, protein powder, and blueberries.

2. Secure the lid and process at high speed until the ingredients are smooth and well combined, 1 to 2 minutes. If unblended ingredients remain or stick to the sides, use a spatula to scrape them down into the blended mixture and continue processing until thoroughly incorporated. The mixture will be a thick liquid.

3. If desired, add the ice to the blender, close the lid, and process on the ice crush setting (or high speed) until the ingredients are smooth and the ice is thoroughly incorporated, 1 to 2 minutes. The smoothie should have a thick consistency.

4. Serve immediately.

Variation Tip: Any berries will suffice. Use whatever you have stashed away in your freezer. Frozen mixed berries work well, too.

Per Serving: Macronutrients: 49% Fat, 36% Protein, 15% Carbs; Calories: 365; Total Fat: 20g; Protein: 33g; Total Carbs: 16g; Fiber: 5g; Net Carbs: 11g

Crunchy Granola Smoothie Bowl

Prep time: 5 minutes | **Yield:** 1 serving | High Fat

If you prefer to sit down for a mindful meal instead of on the go through a straw, smoothie bowls are a great way to enjoy your blended beauties one bite at a time with a spoon. Create designs with garnishes and toppings to transform them into stunning works of art!

1 cup unsweetened cashew milk (or preferred dairy-free milk)

1 teaspoon MCT oil

½ cup fresh or frozen blackberries (or any frozen berry)

1 cup crushed or cubed ice

¼ cup mixed nuts, roughly chopped

2 tablespoons unsweetened dried coconut flakes

1 tablespoon chia seeds

1. In a blender, combine the cashew milk, MCT oil, and blackberries.

2. Secure the lid and process at high speed until the ingredients are smooth and well combined, 1 to 2 minutes. If unblended ingredients remain or stick to the sides, use a spatula to scrape them down into the blended mixture and continue processing until thoroughly incorporated. The mixture will be a thin liquid.

3. Add the ice to the blender, close the lid, and process on the ice crush setting (or high speed) until the ingredients are smooth and the ice is thoroughly incorporated into the mixture, 1 to 2 minutes. The smoothie should have a thick consistency.

4. Pour the mixture into a serving bowl and top with the mixed nuts, coconut flakes, and chia seeds. Serve with a spoon and enjoy immediately.

Variation Tip: Instead of the mixed nuts, try topping the smoothie bowl with a keto-friendly commercial granola blend from brands such as NuTrail, Purely Elizabeth, and Thrive Market.

Per Serving: Macronutrients: 77% Fat, 9% Protein, 14% Carbs; Calories: 431; Total Fat: 37g; Protein: 10g; Total Carbs: 23g; Fiber: 11g; Net Carbs: 12g

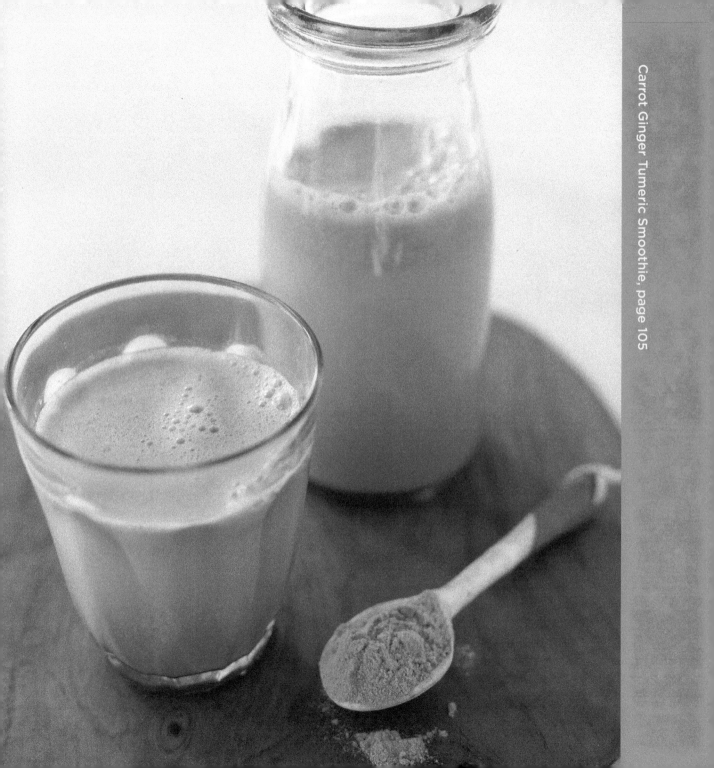

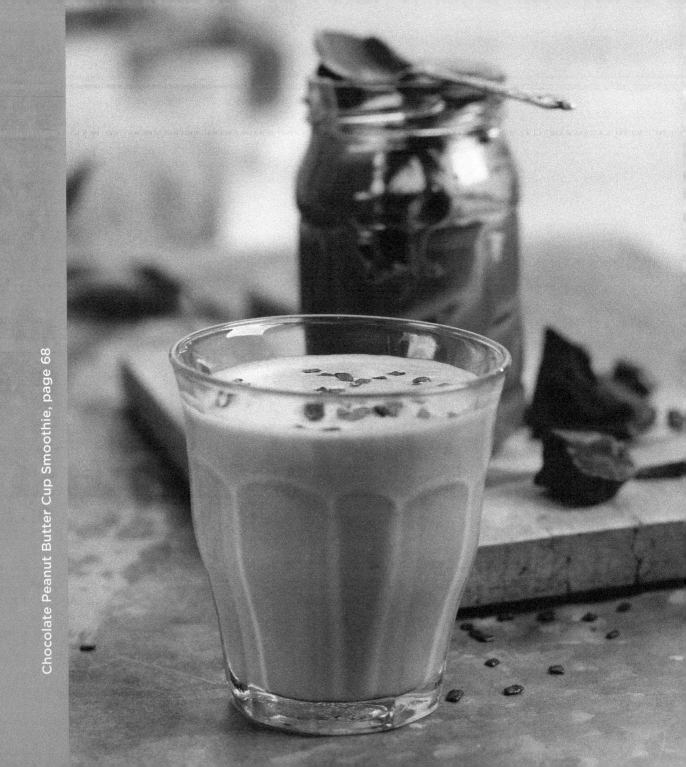

Chocolate Peanut Butter Cup Smoothie, page 68

CHAPTER 4

CHOCOLATY

Insatiable chocolate cravings? I got you. This chapter has a variety of recipes that will satisfy your inner chocoholic without causing you to deviate from your goals. Keto-friendly chocolate options are used to keep the carbs low—cacao nibs, cocoa powder, cocoa powder, and dark chocolate are all featured in this chapter. Whether you prefer the rich flavors of bitter dark chocolate, creamy and sweet milk chocolate, or light and buttery white chocolate, you'll find something to delight your taste buds in the pages that follow.

White Chocolate Protein Shake

Prep time: 5 minutes | **Yield:** 1 serving | High Fat, High Protein, Super Low Carb

This simple smoothie uses cocoa butter, vanilla, and sweetener to imitate the delicate, creamy flavor of white chocolate. A quick scoop of protein powder elevates this recipe from a sweet treat to a filling meal, but feel free to enjoy it as a snack or post-workout shake as well.

1 cup unsweetened macadamia nut milk (or preferred dairy-free milk)

1 teaspoon vanilla extract

1 scoop whey protein isolate powder (or preferred protein powder)

1 teaspoon monkfruit erythritol blend sweetener (or preferred sweetener)

2 tablespoons cocoa butter, melted

1 cup crushed or cubed ice (optional)

1. In a blender, combine the macadamia nut milk, vanilla, protein powder, and sweetener.

2. Secure the lid and process at high speed until the ingredients are well combined, 1 to 2 minutes.

3. While the blender is running, slowly pour in the melted cocoa butter through the opening in the lid to prevent clumping. If unblended ingredients remain or stick to the sides, use a spatula to scrape them down into the blended mixture and continue processing until thoroughly incorporated. The mixture will be a thin liquid.

4. If desired, add the ice to the blender, close the lid, and process on the ice crush setting (or high speed) until the ingredients are smooth and the ice is thoroughly incorporated, 1 to 2 minutes. The smoothie should have a thick, creamy consistency.

5. Serve immediately.

Variation Tip: This protein shake makes an excellent base to build on. Try adding citrus fruit, berries, coconut, or coffee (instant or cold brew).

Per Serving: Macronutrients: 71% Fat, 24% Protein, 5% Carbs; Calories: 433; Total Fat: 34g; Protein: 26g; Total Carbs: 7g; Fiber: 1g; Net Carbs: 2g; Erythritol: 4g

Chocolate Protein Shake

Prep time: 5 minutes | **Yield:** 1 serving | High Fat, High Protein, Super Low Carb

Need a quick chocolate fix? This protein-rich chocolate smoothie is perfect for breakfast on the go or a speedy afternoon snack. You can also enjoy this recipe after your workout as an easy recovery shake. The whey protein provides essential amino acids critical for muscle repair and growth.

1 cup unsweetened macadamia nut milk (or preferred dairy-free milk)

1 tablespoon MCT oil

1 scoop whey protein isolate powder (or preferred protein powder)

1 tablespoon cocoa powder

½ teaspoon monkfruit erythritol blend sweetener or preferred sweetener (optional)

2 tablespoons cacao nibs

1 cup crushed or cubed ice (optional)

1. In a blender, combine the macadamia nut milk, MCT oil, protein powder, cocoa powder, sweetener (if desired), and cacao nibs.

2. Secure the lid and process at high speed until the ingredients are smooth and well combined, 1 to 2 minutes. If unblended ingredients remain or stick to the sides, use a spatula to scrape them down into the blended mixture and continue processing until thoroughly incorporated. The mixture will be a thin liquid.

3. If desired, add the ice to the blender, close the lid, and process on the ice crush setting (or high speed) until the ingredients are smooth and the ice is thoroughly incorporated, 1 to 2 minutes. The smoothie should have a thick consistency.

4. Serve immediately.

Per Serving: Macronutrients: 65% Fat, 25% Protein, 10% Carbs; Calories: 429; Total Fat: 31g; Protein: 27g; Total Carbs: 14g; Fiber: 9g; Net Carbs: 3g; Erythritol: 2g

White Chocolate Macadamia Nut Smoothie

Prep time: 5 minutes | **Yield:** 1 serving | High Fat, High Protein, Super Low Carb

If you're hunting for a filling recipe, look no further. The high protein and fat content of this smoothie will leave you full and content all morning long. Plus it's delicious! Cocoa butter and vanilla are blended into ultra-creamy macadamia nut milk for a silky-smooth white chocolate flavor that's highlighted with rich, buttery macadamia nuts and cinnamon spice.

1 cup unsweetened macadamia nut milk

1 teaspoon vanilla extract

1 scoop whey protein isolate powder (or preferred protein powder)

½ teaspoon ground cinnamon

2 tablespoons macadamia nuts

2 tablespoons cocoa butter, melted

1 cup crushed or cubed ice (optional)

1. In a blender, combine the macadamia nut milk, vanilla, protein powder, cinnamon, and macadamia nuts.

2. Secure the lid and process at high speed until the ingredients are well combined, 1 to 2 minutes.

3. While the blender is running, slowly pour in the melted cocoa butter through the opening in the lid to prevent clumping. If unblended ingredients remain or stick to the sides, use a spatula to scrape them down into the blended mixture and continue processing until thoroughly incorporated. The mixture will be a thin liquid.

4. If desired, add the ice to the blender, close the lid, and process on the ice crush setting (or high speed) until the ingredients are smooth and the ice is thoroughly incorporated, 1 to 2 minutes. The smoothie should have a thick, creamy consistency.

5. Serve immediately.

Variation Tip: Consider using almonds, hazelnuts, or a medley of mixed nuts for variety.

Per Serving: Macronutrients: 76% Fat, 19% Protein, 5% Carbs; Calories: 556; Total Fat: 47g; Protein: 27g; Total Carbs: 7g; Fiber: 3g; Net Carbs: 4g

Chocolate Coconut Cream Smoothie

Prep time: 5 minutes | **Yield:** 1 serving | High Fat, Super Low Carb

This smoothie had me at first sip. The creamy dark chocolate contrasted with the sweet coconut milk creates a flavor combination that's out of this world. Though it might taste indulgent, this recipe is rich in micronutrients and totally keto-compliant.

1 cup unsweetened coconut milk beverage

¼ cup plus 2 tablespoons unsweetened coconut cream

1 tablespoon unsweetened cocoa powder

½ teaspoon monkfruit erythritol blend sweetener (or preferred sweetener)

2 tablespoons cacao nibs

1 cup crushed or cubed ice (optional)

1. In a blender, combine the coconut milk beverage, coconut cream, cocoa powder, sweetener, and cacao nibs.

2. Secure the lid and process at high speed until the ingredients are smooth and well combined, 1 to 2 minutes. If unblended ingredients remain or stick to the sides, use a spatula to scrape them down into the blended mixture and continue processing until thoroughly incorporated. The mixture will be a thick liquid.

3. If desired, add the ice to the blender, close the lid, and process on the ice crush setting (or high speed) until the ingredients are smooth and the ice is thoroughly incorporated, 1 to 2 minutes. The smoothie should have a thick, creamy consistency.

4. Serve immediately.

Variation Tip: Unsweetened coconut flakes can be blended in directly to develop the texture or sprinkled on top for a delicate garnish.

Per Serving: Macronutrients: 82% Fat, 2% Protein, 16% Carbs; Calories: 362; Total Fat: 33g; Protein: 2g; Total Carbs: 14g; Fiber: 8g; Net Carbs: 4g; Erythritol: 2g

German Chocolate Cake Shake

Prep time: 5 minutes | **Yield:** 1 serving | High Fat, Super Low Carb

German chocolate cake appears at my family gatherings several times a year. It's Mom's favorite, after all! The ingredients go so well together; why not blend them up in a smoothie? Decadent, buttery chocolate, coconut, and pecans—without the sugar rush!

1 cup unsweetened coconut milk beverage

1 teaspoon vanilla extract

2 tablespoons unsweetened cocoa powder

1 teaspoon erythritol brown sugar replacement (or preferred sweetener)

Pinch sea salt

¼ cup pecans

2 tablespoons unsweetened dried coconut flakes

1 tablespoon butter or ghee, melted and slightly cooled

1 cup crushed or cubed ice (optional)

1. In a blender, combine the coconut milk beverage, vanilla, cocoa powder, sweetener, sea salt, pecans, and coconut flakes.

2. Secure the lid and process at high speed until the ingredients are well combined, 1 to 2 minutes.

3. While the blender is running, slowly pour in the melted butter through the opening in the lid to prevent clumping. If unblended ingredients remain or stick to the sides, use a spatula to scrape them down into the blended mixture and continue processing until thoroughly incorporated. The consistency will be a thick liquid.

4. If desired, add the ice to the blender, close the lid, and process on high until the ingredients are smooth and the ice is thoroughly incorporated into the mixture, 1 to 2 minutes. The smoothie should have a thick, fluffy consistency.

5. Serve immediately.

Variation Tip: Blend in ¼ to ½ cup of plain Greek yogurt to boost the creaminess and protein content and balance out the sweetness of the smoothie with a subtle, pleasant tang.

Per Serving: Macronutrients: 91% Fat, 5% Protein, 4% Carbs; Calories: 436; Total Fat: 44g; Protein: 6g; Total Carbs: 18g; Fiber: g; Net Carbs: 5g; Erythritol: 4g

Mint Chocolate Chip Smoothie

Prep time: 5 minutes | **Yield:** 1 serving | High Fat, Super Low Carb

I'm a sucker for anything mint and chocolate. Who doesn't love cool, refreshing mint flavors balanced with delightful sweetness? I couldn't resist making a keto-friendly mint chocolate chip smoothie. This drink is the perfect way to satisfy a sweet tooth without all the sugar.

1 cup unsweetened almond milk (or preferred dairy-free milk)

2 tablespoons heavy (whipping) cream

½ teaspoon vanilla extract

½ teaspoon monkfruit erythritol blend sweetener (or preferred sweetener)

½ avocado, peeled, pitted, and cut into chunks

¼ cup fresh mint leaves

2 tablespoons cacao nibs

1 cup crushed or cubed ice (optional)

1. In a blender, combine the almond milk, heavy cream, vanilla, sweetener, avocado, mint, and cacao nibs.

2. Secure the lid and process at high speed until the ingredients are smooth and well combined, 1 to 2 minutes. If unblended ingredients remain or stick to the sides, use a spatula to scrape them down into the blended mixture and continue processing until thoroughly incorporated. The mixture will be a thick liquid.

3. If desired, add the ice to the blender, close the lid, and process on the ice crush setting (or high speed) until the ingredients are smooth and the ice is thoroughly incorporated into the mixture, 1 to 2 minutes. The smoothie should have a thick, creamy consistency.

4. Serve immediately.

Per Serving: Macronutrients: 78% Fat, 3% Protein, Carbs; Calories: 381; Total Fat: 33g; Protein: 3g; Total Carbs: 19g; Fiber: 12g; Net Carbs: 5g; Erythritol: 2g

Net Carbs
6g

White Chocolate Raspberry Cream Smoothie

Prep time: 5 minutes | **Yield:** 1 serving | High Fat, Super Low Carb

This recipe is a must-have for summer, when fresh raspberries abound. Its light, fluffy goodness is perfect for cooling down on hot days or after an intense workout session. Rich white chocolate flavor and heavy cream amplify the sweetness of the raspberries, creating a perfect balance in every sip.

⅔ cup cold water

⅓ cup heavy (whipping) cream

1 teaspoon vanilla extract

1 teaspoon monkfruit erythritol blend sweetener (or preferred sweetener)

½ cup fresh or frozen raspberries

2 tablespoons cocoa butter, melted

1 cup crushed or cubed ice (optional)

1. In a blender, combine the water, heavy cream, vanilla, sweetener, and raspberries.
2. Secure the lid and process at high speed until the ingredients are well combined, 1 to 2 minutes.
3. While the blender is running, slowly pour in the melted cocoa butter through the opening in the lid to prevent clumping. If unblended ingredients remain or stick to the sides, use a spatula to scrape them down into the blended mixture and continue processing until thoroughly incorporated. The mixture will be a thin, creamy liquid.
4. If desired, add the ice to the blender, close the lid, and process on the ice crush setting (or high speed) until the ingredients are smooth and the ice is thoroughly incorporated, 1 to 2 minutes. The smoothie should have a thick, creamy consistency.
5. Serve immediately.

Variation Tip: Blackberries, strawberries, blueberries, or huckleberries would be a fantastic swap or addition.

Per Serving: Macronutrients: 91% Fat, 2% Protein, 7% Carbs; Calories: 552; Total Fat: 56g; Protein: 3g; Total Carbs: 14g; Fiber: 4g; Net Carbs: 6g; Erythritol: 4g

Chocolate Avocado Smoothie

Prep time: 5 minutes | **Yield:** 1 serving | High Fat, Super Low Carb

Here's another chocolate treat you can feel good about! Not only is this smoothie chocolaty, creamy, and keto-friendly, but also it delivers a lot of nutritional benefits. Thanks to the avocado, it's loaded with vitamins, minerals, and antioxidants. It's also rich in fiber and healthy fats that help keep you fuller for longer.

1 cup unsweetened almond milk (or preferred dairy-free milk)

1 tablespoon avocado oil

1 tablespoon unsweetened
 cocoa powder

½ teaspoon monkfruit erythritol blend
 sweetener (or preferred sweetener)

1 avocado, peeled, pitted, and cut
 into chunks

1 cup crushed or cubed ice (optional)

1. In a blender, combine the almond milk, avocado oil, cocoa powder, sweetener, and avocado.

2. Secure the lid and process at high speed until the ingredients are smooth and well combined, 1 to 2 minutes. If unblended ingredients remain or stick to the sides, use a spatula to scrape them down into the blended mixture and continue processing until thoroughly incorporated. The mixture will be a thick liquid.

3. If desired, add the ice to the blender, close the lid, and process on the ice crush setting (or high speed) until the ingredients are smooth and the ice is thoroughly incorporated, 1 to 2 minutes. The smoothie should have a thick, creamy consistency.

4. Serve immediately.

Variation Tip: Consider adding banana flavor extract to mimic the flavor of a banana mix-in.

Per Serving: Macronutrients: 86% Fat, 5% Protein, 9% Carbs; Calories: 396; Total Fat: 38g; Protein: 5g; Total Carbs: 20g; Fiber: 12g; Net Carbs: 6g; Erythritol: 2g

Candy Bar Smoothie Bowl

Prep time: 5 minutes | **Yield:** 1 serving | High Protein, Super Low Carb

You may have thought candy bars were a thing of the past. You can't have candy bars on keto, right? Wrong! I do believe this smoothie recipe proves otherwise. The flavors are inspired by my favorite non-keto treat: Snickers. Peanuts add a wonderful crunchy texture to contrast the rich, creamy chocolate.

1 cup unsweetened almond milk (or preferred dairy-free milk)

2 tablespoons unsweetened powdered peanut butter (also called peanut powder or peanut flour)

2 tablespoons collagen hydrolysate powder

1 tablespoon unsweetened cocoa powder

½ teaspoon monkfruit erythritol blend sweetener (or preferred sweetener)

1 cup crushed or cubed ice

2 tablespoons peanuts, chopped, for garnish

2 tablespoons cacao nibs, for garnish

1. In a blender, combine the almond milk, powdered peanut butter, collagen powder, cocoa powder, and sweetener.

2. Secure the lid and process at high speed until the ingredients are smooth and well combined, 1 to 2 minutes. If unblended ingredients remain or stick to the sides, use a spatula to scrape them down into the blended mixture and continue processing until thoroughly incorporated. The mixture will be a thin liquid.

3. Add the ice to the blender, close the lid, and process on the ice crush setting (or high speed) until the ingredients are smooth and the ice is thoroughly incorporated into the mixture, 1 to 2 minutes. The smoothie should have a thick, fluffy consistency.

4. Pour the mixture into a serving bowl and top with the peanuts and cacao nibs. Enjoy immediately.

Per Serving: Macronutrients: 58% Fat, 26% Protein, 16% Carbs; Calories: 370; Total Fat: 24g; Protein: 24g; Total Carbs: 20g; Fiber: 12g; Net Carbs: 6g; Erythritol: 2g

Fudge Pop Smoothie

Prep time: 5 minutes | **Yield:** 1 serving | High Fat, Super Low Carb

When the weather warms up, frozen fudge pops are a summertime favorite. The traditional ones are unquestionably delicious; they're also loaded with sugar. This creamy, chocolaty smoothie is a perfect keto-friendly substitute that'll satisfy the craving. You can even use the base to mold your own frozen treats!

½ **cup heavy (whipping) cream**

½ **cup unsweetened cashew milk (or preferred nut milk)**

½ **teaspoon vanilla extract**

2 **tablespoons unsweetened cocoa powder**

1 **teaspoon monkfruit erythritol blend sweetener (or preferred sweetener)**

1 **cup crushed or cubed ice**

1. In a blender, combine the heavy cream, cashew milk, vanilla, cocoa powder, and sweetener.

2. Secure the lid and process at high speed until the ingredients are smooth and well combined, 1 to 2 minutes. If unblended ingredients remain or stick to the sides, use a spatula to scrape them down into the blended mixture and continue processing until thoroughly incorporated. The mixture will be a thin liquid.

3. Add the ice to the blender, close the lid, and process on the ice crush setting (or high speed) until the ingredients are smooth and the ice is thoroughly incorporated into the mixture, 1 to 2 minutes. The smoothie should have a thick, creamy consistency.

4. Serve immediately.

Per Serving: Macronutrients: 90% Fat, 5% Protein, 5% Carbs; Calories: 448; Total Fat: 45g; Protein: 6g; Total Carbs: 15g; Fiber: 4g; Net Carbs: 7g; Erythritol: 4g

Dark Chocolate Blueberry Smoothie

Prep time: 5 minutes | **Yield:** 1 serving | High Fat, Super Low Carb

Sweet berries are one of my favorite ways to balance the bitterness of dark chocolate. Here, we'll pair blueberries with keto-friendly baking chips or cacao nibs, the light pop of fruit balancing the deep, rich chocolate flavors.

1 cup macadamia nut milk (or preferred dairy-free milk)

2 tablespoons MCT oil

½ teaspoon ground cinnamon

Pinch sea salt

1 ounce keto-friendly dark chocolate baking chips (such as Lily's) or cacao nibs

¼ cup fresh or frozen blueberries

1 cup crushed or cubed ice (optional)

1. In a blender, combine the macadamia nut milk, MCT oil, cinnamon, sea salt, chocolate chips, and blueberries.

2. Secure the lid and process at high speed until the ingredients are smooth and well combined, 1 to 2 minutes. If unblended ingredients remain or stick to the sides, use a spatula to scrape them down into the blended mixture and continue processing until thoroughly incorporated. The mixture will be a thin liquid.

3. If desired, add the ice to the blender, close the lid, and process on the ice crush setting (or high speed) until the ingredients are smooth and the ice is thoroughly incorporated, 1 to 2 minutes. The smoothie should have a thick, fluffy consistency.

4. Serve immediately.

Variation Tip: Boost the chocolate flavor even more with a teaspoon of unsweetened cocoa powder.

Per Serving: Macronutrients: 88% Fat, 3% Protein, 9% Carbs; Calories: 428; Total Fat: 42g; Protein: 3g; Total Carbs: 24g; Fiber: 11g; Net Carbs: 7g; Erythritol: 6g

Chocolate Peanut Butter Cup Smoothie

Prep time: 5 minutes | **Yield:** 1 serving | High Protein, Super Low Carb

What's better than a chocolate peanut butter shake? A low-carb, keto-friendly chocolate peanut butter shake! Rich, creamy, and thick, this sugar-free recipe tastes like a blended-up peanut butter cup. It's a perfect breakfast or snack to help keep you on track with your goals.

1 cup macadamia nut milk (or preferred nut milk)

2 tablespoons unsweetened natural peanut butter

1 tablespoon unsweetened cocoa powder

½ teaspoon monkfruit erythritol blend sweetener (or preferred sweetener)

1 scoop whey protein isolate powder (or preferred protein powder)

1 cup crushed or cubed ice (optional)

1. In a blender, combine the macadamia nut milk, peanut butter, cocoa powder, sweetener, and protein powder.

2. Secure the lid and process at high speed until the ingredients are smooth and well combined, 1 to 2 minutes. If unblended ingredients remain or stick to the sides, use a spatula to scrape them down into the blended mixture and continue processing until thoroughly incorporated. The mixture will be a thin liquid.

3. If desired, add the ice to the blender, close the lid, and process on the ice crush setting (or high speed) until the ingredients are smooth and the ice is thoroughly incorporated, 1 to 2 minutes. The smoothie should have a thick, fluffy consistency.

4. Serve immediately.

Variation Tip: Swap in (or add some) unsweetened powdered peanut butter to boost the flavor and protein without spiking the calorie content.

Per Serving: Macronutrients: 56% Fat, 35% Protein, 9% Carbs; Calories: 385; Total Fat: 24g; Protein: 34g; Total Carbs: 15g; Fiber: 5g; Net Carbs: 8g; Erythritol: 2g

Chocolate Almond Coconut Shake

Prep time: 5 minutes | **Yield:** 1 serving | High Fat, High Protein, Super Low Carb

Cocoa powder provides a dark-chocolaty base, while almond and coconut enhance the flavor and texture. Imagine an Almond Joy candy bar blended up into a shake without all the sugar and carbs, and you'd be right on the money with this delicious smoothie.

1 cup unsweetened almond milk (or coconut milk beverage)

2 tablespoons almond butter

2 tablespoons collagen hydrolysate powder

1 tablespoon unsweetened cocoa powder

1 teaspoon monkfruit erythritol blend sweetener (or preferred sweetener)

Pinch sea salt

¼ cup unsweetened dried coconut flakes

1 cup crushed or cubed ice (optional)

1. In a blender, combine the almond milk, almond butter, collagen powder, cocoa powder, sweetener, sea salt, and coconut flakes.

2. Secure the lid and process at high speed until the ingredients are smooth and well combined, 1 to 2 minutes. If unblended ingredients remain or stick to the sides, use a spatula to scrape them down into the blended mixture and continue processing until thoroughly incorporated. The mixture will be a thick liquid.

3. If desired, add the ice to the blender, close the lid, and process on the ice crush setting (or high speed) until the ingredients are smooth and the ice is thoroughly incorporated into the mixture, 1 to 2 minutes. The smoothie should have a thick, fluffy consistency.

4. Serve immediately.

Per Serving: Macronutrients: 72% Fat, 21% Protein, 7% Carbs; Calories: 415; Total Fat: 33g; Protein: 22g; Total Carbs: 21g; Fiber: 9g; Net Carbs: 8g; Erythritol: 4g

Chocolate Cauliflower Smoothie

Prep time: 5 minutes | **Yield:** 1 serving | High Fat, Super Low Carb

Chocolate and cauliflower may seem like an odd combo, but it really works. Chocolate remains the true star of the show; the frozen cauliflower serves to enhance nutrition and texture in this smoothie, providing a lush creaminess without overpowering the sharp, rich flavor of the cocoa powder.

1 cup unsweetened almond milk (or preferred dairy-free milk)

2 tablespoons MCT oil

2 tablespoons unsweetened cocoa powder

½ teaspoon monkfruit erythritol blend sweetener or preferred sweetener (optional)

Pinch sea salt

1 cup chopped or riced frozen cauliflower

1. In a blender, combine the almond milk, MCT oil, cocoa powder, sweetener (if desired), and sea salt.

2. Secure the lid and process at high speed until the ingredients are smooth and well combined, 1 to 2 minutes. If unblended ingredients remain or stick to the sides, use a spatula to scrape them down into the blended mixture and continue processing until thoroughly incorporated. The mixture will be a thin liquid.

3. Add the frozen cauliflower to the blender, close the lid, and process on the ice crush setting (or high speed) until the ingredients are smooth and the cauliflower is thoroughly incorporated, 1 to 2 minutes. The smoothie should have a thick, fluffy consistency.

4. Serve immediately.

Variation Tip: A tablespoon or two of nut or seed butter will boost the fat content and add a welcome nutty flavor.

Per Serving: Macronutrients: 90% Fat, 8% Protein, 2% Carbs; Calories: 320; Total Fat: 32g; Protein: 6g; Total Carbs: 17g; Fiber: 7g; Net Carbs: 8g; Erythritol: 2g

Blended Iced Mocha Smoothie

Prep time: 5 minutes | **Yield:** 1 serving | High Fat

If you start your day with a trip to the barista, I hereby present you with a healthier option. This low-carb mocha smoothie contains the traditional coffee and chocolate flavor combo we all know and love. It's perfect for anyone who wants a delicious caffeinated treat without all the sugar!

¾ cup unsweetened almond milk (or preferred dairy-free milk)

¼ cup heavy (whipping) cream

2 tablespoons instant coffee powder

1 tablespoon unsweetened cocoa powder

1 teaspoon monkfruit erythritol blend sweetener (or preferred sweetener)

1 cup crushed or cubed ice

2 tablespoons unsweetened whipped cream, for garnish (optional)

1 tablespoon cacao nibs, for garnish (optional)

1. In a blender, combine the almond milk, heavy cream, coffee powder, cocoa powder, and sweetener.

2. Secure the lid and process at high speed until the ingredients are smooth and well combined, 1 to 2 minutes. If unblended ingredients remain or stick to the sides, use a spatula to scrape them down into the blended mixture and continue processing until thoroughly incorporated. The mixture will be a thin liquid.

3. Add the ice, close the lid, and process on the ice crush setting (or high speed) until the ingredients are smooth and the ice is thoroughly incorporated, 1 to 2 minutes. The smoothie should have a thick, fluffy, creamy consistency.

4. Pour the mixture into a serving glass. Top with the whipped cream and garnish with cacao nibs, if desired. Enjoy immediately.

Variation Tip: Make this a blended pumpkin spice latte! Just swap out the cocoa powder and cacao nibs for a tablespoon or two of pumpkin puree and a teaspoon of pumpkin pie spice.

Per Serving: Macronutrients: 82% Fat, 6% Protein, 12% Carbs; Calories: 264; Total Fat: 24g; Protein: 4g; Total Carbs: 16g; Fiber: 2g; Net Carbs: 10g; Erythritol: 4g

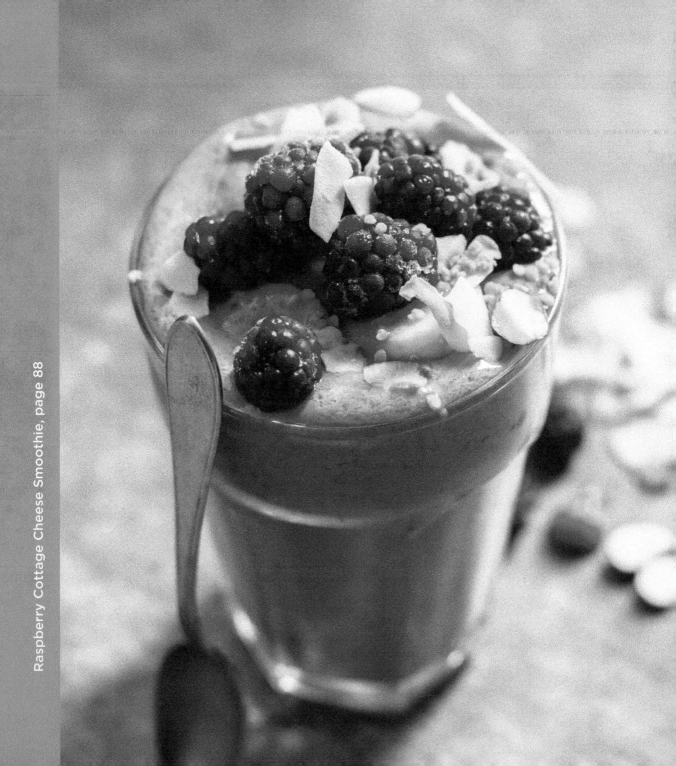

Raspberry Cottage Cheese Smoothie, page 88

CHAPTER 5

FRUITY

Fruit-filled drinks are standard smoothie fare; however, fruity recipes low in sugar and carbs are much harder to track down. I'm happy to report that the recipes in this chapter are devoted to fruity shakes and smoothies with keto-friendly macros and ingredients. Berries, avocado, citrus, and coconut are the stars of the show within the following pages. You'll come across sweet dessertlike goodies, protein-packed shakes, and frosty blended spritzers to sip and savor throughout the day. In this chapter, you'll learn the best ways to incorporate fruit into your keto smoothie repertoire with mouthwatering recipes that will double as inspiration for your own unique creations.

Coconut Vanilla Lemongrass Tea Smoothie

Prep time: 5 minutes | **Yield:** 1 serving | High Fat, Super Low Carb

In this recipe, sweet, creamy coconut and vanilla pair with citrusy lemongrass for a fresh tropical treat. Lemongrass tea is used to deliver the pleasant lemony flavor instead of the tough, fibrous lemongrass herb to improve blending and ensure the texture is silky smooth.

1 cup lemongrass tea, brewed and chilled
½ cup unsweetened coconut cream
1 teaspoon vanilla extract

¼ cup unsweetened dried coconut flakes
1 cup crushed or cubed ice (optional)

1. In a blender, combine the lemongrass tea, coconut cream, vanilla, and coconut flakes.

2. Secure the lid and process at high speed until the ingredients are smooth and well combined, 1 to 2 minutes. If unblended ingredients remain or stick to the sides, use a spatula to scrape them down into the blended mixture and continue processing until thoroughly incorporated. The mixture will be a thick liquid.

3. If desired, add the ice to the blender, close the lid, and process on the ice crush setting (or high speed) until the ingredients are smooth and the ice is thoroughly incorporated, 1 to 2 minutes. The smoothie should have a thick, creamy consistency.

4. Serve immediately.

Per Serving: Macronutrients: 86% Fat, 1% Protein, 13% Carbs; Calories: 385; Total Fat: 37g; Protein: 1g; Total Carbs: 7g; Fiber: 3g; Net Carbs: 4g

Coconut Key Lime Cheesecake

Prep time: 5 minutes | **Yield:** 1 serving | High Fat, Super Low Carb

Who says you can't have dessert for breakfast? This decadent smoothie is like a slice of cheesecake in a glass, complete with a keto-friendly "graham cracker" crust topping. The freshly squeezed lime juice adds a bright, tangy sweetness, reminiscent of key lime pie.

½ **cup cold water**

¼ **cup unsweetened coconut cream**

Juice of ½ lime

¼ **cup (2 ounces) cream cheese, softened**

1⅛ **teaspoons powdered erythritol or allulose sweetener (or preferred sweetener), divided**

1 **cup crushed or cubed ice (optional)**

1 **teaspoon almond flour**

⅛ **teaspoon ground cinnamon**

1. In a blender, combine the water, coconut cream, lime juice, cream cheese, and 1 teaspoon of sweetener.

2. Secure the lid and process at high speed until the ingredients are smooth and well combined, 1 to 2 minutes. If unblended ingredients remain or stick to the sides, use a spatula to scrape them down into the blended mixture and continue processing until thoroughly incorporated. The mixture will be a thick liquid.

3. If desired, add the ice to the blender, close the lid, and process at high speed until smooth and thoroughly incorporated, 1 to 2 minutes. The smoothie should have a thick, fluffy consistency.

4. Pour the mixture into a serving glass. Combine the remaining ⅛ teaspoon of sweetener, the almond flour, and cinnamon in a small dish; then sprinkle over the top of the prepared smoothie.

Variation Tip: To trim the carbs even further, swap out the lime juice for lemon juice, or omit the citrus altogether.

Per Serving: Macronutrients: 88% Fat, 5% Protein, 7% Carbs; Calories: 338; Total Fat: 33g; Protein: 4g; Total Carbs: 10g; Fiber: 1g; Net Carbs: 5g; Erythritol: 4g

Maple Ginger Strawberry Rhubarb Smoothie

Prep time: 5 minutes | **Yield:** 1 serving | Super Low Carb

Raw rhubarb is tart on its own, but strawberries and erythritol balance things nicely with their sweetness. Ginger and maple supply a warm, spicy kick with notes of caramel.

1 cup cold water

2 tablespoons MCT oil

1 teaspoon maple extract

1 teaspoon erythritol brown sugar replacement (or preferred sweetener)

½ teaspoon ground ginger

½ cup fresh or frozen strawberries

½ stalk fresh or frozen fresh rhubarb, cut into 1-inch pieces

1 cup crushed or cubed ice (optional)

1. In a blender, combine the water, MCT oil, maple extract, sweetener, ginger, strawberries, and rhubarb.

2. Secure the lid and process at high speed until the ingredients are smooth and well combined, 1 to 2 minutes. If unblended ingredients remain or stick to the sides, use a spatula to scrape them down into the blended mixture and continue processing until thoroughly incorporated. The mixture will be a thick liquid.

3. If desired, add the ice to the blender, close the lid, and process on the ice crush setting (or high speed) until the ingredients are smooth and the ice is thoroughly incorporated, 1 to 2 minutes. The smoothie should have a thick, fluffy consistency.

4. Serve immediately.

Variation Tip: If you prefer the milder flavor of cooked rhubarb, you can prepare a compote instead of using the raw vegetable. Just combine chopped rhubarb with sweetener and ¼ cup of water in a small saucepan and bring to a boil over medium heat. Cook until the rhubarb softens and the liquid reduces, 5 to 6 minutes.

Per Serving: Macronutrients: 95% Fat, 2% Protein, 7% Carbs; Calories: 265; Total Fat: 28g; Protein: 1g; Total Carbs: 12g; Fiber: 2g; Net Carbs: 6g; Erythritol: 4g

Strawberry Italian Cream Soda Smoothie

Prep time: 5 minutes | **Yield:** 1 serving | High Fat, Super Low Carb

Love the effervescence of sparkling water? Try it as the liquid base in your smoothie! The signature fizz adds a surprising texture that works wonderfully with fruit flavors.

1 cup strawberry or unflavored unsweet- ened sparkling water

¼ cup heavy (whipping) cream

1 tablespoon MCT oil

½ teaspoon monkfruit erythritol blend sweetener (or preferred sweetener)

½ cup fresh or frozen strawberries

1 cup crushed or cubed ice (optional)

1. In a blender, combine the sparkling water, heavy cream, MCT oil, sweetener, and strawberries.

2. Secure the lid and process at high speed until the ingredients are smooth and well combined, 1 to 2 minutes. If unblended ingredients remain or stick to the sides, use a spatula to scrape them down into the blended mixture and continue processing until thoroughly incorporated. The mixture will be a thick liquid.

3. If desired, add the ice to the blender, close the lid, and process on the ice crush setting (or high speed) until the ingredients are smooth and the ice is thoroughly incorporated, 1 to 2 minutes. The smoothie should have a thick, creamy consistency.

4. Serve immediately.

Per Serving: Macronutrients: 94% Fat, 2% Protein, 4% Carbs; Calories: 343; Total Fat: 36g; Protein: 2g; Total Carbs: 10g; Fiber: 2g; Net Carbs: 6g; Erythritol: 2g

Sparkling Blackberry Spritzer Smoothie

Prep time: 5 minutes | **Yield:** 1 serving | High Fat, Super Low Carb

Fizzy smoothies are so much fun and make the perfect refresher for hot weather. I enjoy combining the fruit-flavored sparkling waters with their fresh or frozen counterparts for a sweet treat—berries are the ideal keto-friendly option.

1 cup blackberry or unflavored unsweetened sparkling water

3 tablespoons MCT oil

1 teaspoon vanilla extract

½ teaspoon monkfruit erythritol blend sweetener (or preferred sweetener)

1 cup fresh or frozen blackberries

1 cup crushed or cubed ice (optional)

1. In a blender, combine the sparkling water, MCT oil, vanilla, sweetener, and blackberries.

2. Secure the lid and process at high speed until the ingredients are smooth and well combined, 1 to 2 minutes. If unblended ingredients remain or stick to the sides, use a spatula to scrape them down into the blended mixture and continue processing until thoroughly incorporated. The mixture will be a thick liquid.

3. If desired, add the ice to the blender, close the lid, and process on the ice crush setting (or high speed) until the ingredients are smooth and the ice is thoroughly incorporated, 1 to 2 minutes. The smoothie should have a thick, fluffy consistency.

4. Serve immediately.

Variation Tip: Switch things up with different berry combinations. Strawberries and raspberries are exceptional paired with their respective flavored sparkling waters.

Per Serving: Macronutrients: 91% Fat, 1% Protein, 5% Carbs; Calories: 423; Total Fat: 43g; Protein: 2g; Total Carbs: 16g; Fiber: 8g; Net Carbs: 6g; Erythritol: 2g

Strawberry Gingersnap Smoothie

Prep time: 5 minutes | **Yield:** 1 serving | High Fat, High Protein, Super Low Carb

Cinnamon, ginger, and cloves create a spicy trifecta balanced by sweet, succulent strawberries in this cookie-inspired smoothie recipe. Protein powder and MCT oil raise the energy and nutritional content for a filling breakfast or post-workout shake.

1 cup cold water

2 tablespoons MCT oil

1 scoop whey protein isolate powder (or preferred protein powder)

1 teaspoon erythritol brown sugar replacement (or preferred sweetener)

½ teaspoon ground cinnamon

½ teaspoon ground ginger

¼ teaspoon ground cloves

½ cup fresh or frozen strawberries

1 cup crushed or cubed ice

1. In a blender, combine the water, MCT oil, protein powder, sweetener, cinnamon, ginger, cloves, and strawberries.

2. Secure the lid and process at high speed until the ingredients are smooth and well combined, 1 to 2 minutes. If unblended ingredients remain or stick to the sides, use a spatula to scrape them down into the blended mixture and continue processing until thoroughly incorporated. The mixture will be a thick liquid.

3. Add the ice to the blender, close the lid, and process on the ice crush setting (or high speed) until the ingredients are smooth and the ice is thoroughly incorporated, 1 to 2 minutes. The smoothie should have a thick, fluffy consistency.

4. Serve immediately.

Per Serving: Macronutrients: 68% Fat, 26% Protein, 6% Carbs; Calories: 395; Total Fat: 30g; Protein: 26g; Total Carbs: 15g; Fiber: 3g; Net Carbs: 8g; Erythritol: 4g

Lemon Lime Avocado Smoothie

Prep time: 5 minutes | **Yield:** 1 serving | High Fat, High Protein, Super Low Carb

Avocados are an unbeatable smoothie upgrade—they simultaneously transform your drink into a nutritional dynamo while producing a lush, silken texture. Plus they go with everything! This smoothie is full of nourishing fats and protein to sustain fullness in between meals.

1 cup cold water

Juice of ½ lemon

Juice of ½ lime

1 tablespoon avocado oil

1 scoop whey protein isolate powder (or preferred protein powder)

½ teaspoon monkfruit erythritol blend sweetener or preferred sweetener (optional)

1 avocado, peeled, pitted, and cut into chunks

1 cup crushed or cubed ice (optional)

1. In a blender, combine the water, lemon juice, lime juice, avocado oil, protein powder, sweetener (if desired), and avocado.

2. Secure the lid and process at high speed until the ingredients are smooth and well combined, 1 to 2 minutes. If unblended ingredients remain or stick to the sides, use a spatula to scrape them down into the blended mixture and continue processing until thoroughly incorporated. The mixture will be a thick liquid.

3. If desired, add the ice to the blender, close the lid, and process on the ice crush setting (or high speed) until the ingredients are smooth and the ice is thoroughly incorporated, 1 to 2 minutes. The smoothie should have a thick, fluffy consistency.

4. Serve immediately.

Variation Tip: Give this drink a tropical twist by swapping the water for coconut milk.

Per Serving: Macronutrients: 68% Fat, 23% Protein, 9% Carbs; Calories: 489; Total Fat: 37g; Protein: 28g; Total Carbs: 19g; Fiber: 9g; Net Carbs: 8g; Erythritol: 2g

Blackberry Mint Zucchini Smoothie

Prep time: 5 minutes | **Yield:** 1 serving | Super Low Carb

This recipe teams up two of my favorite things: fruit and vegetables. The sweetness from the blackberries balances the earthy, "green" flavor, and the zucchini contributes a remarkable creamy texture to the drink.

1 cup unsweetened spearmint tea, brewed and chilled

2 tablespoons MCT oil

1 small zucchini, cut into chunks

¾ cup fresh or frozen blackberries

¼ cup fresh mint leaves

1 cup crushed or cubed ice (optional)

1. In a blender, combine the spearmint tea, MCT oil, zucchini, blackberries, and mint leaves.

2. Secure the lid and process at high speed until the ingredients are smooth and well combined, 1 to 2 minutes. If unblended ingredients remain or stick to the sides, use a spatula to scrape them down into the blended mixture and continue processing until thoroughly incorporated. The mixture will be a thick liquid.

3. If desired, add the ice to the blender, close the lid, and process on the ice crush setting (or high speed) until the ingredients are smooth and the ice is thoroughly incorporated into the mixture. The smoothie should have a thick, fluffy consistency.

4. Serve immediately.

Per Serving: Macronutrients: 85% Fat, 4% Protein, 11% Carbs; Calories: 306; Total Fat: 29g; Protein: 3g; Total Carbs: 16g; Fiber: 7g; Net Carbs: 9g

Lemon Citrus Lassi Protein Smoothie

Prep time: 5 minutes | **Yield:** 1 serving | High Fat, High Protein, Super Low Carb

This recipe is influenced by one of my favorite blended drinks, mango lassi, which is essentially a yogurt-based smoothie. High-sugar mango is traded for low-sugar citrus, and keto-friendly sweetener replaces the standard sugar. Protein powder and MCT oil boost the energy and nutritional content, making it a full meal.

½ **cup cold water**

½ **cup plain full-fat Greek yogurt**

Juice of 1 lemon

2 tablespoons MCT oil

1 scoop whey protein isolate powder (or preferred protein powder)

½ **teaspoon monkfruit erythritol blend sweetener (or preferred sweetener)**

1 cup crushed or cubed ice

1. In a blender, combine the water, Greek yogurt, lemon juice, MCT oil, protein powder, and sweetener.

2. Secure the lid and process at high speed until the ingredients are smooth and well combined, 1 to 2 minutes. If unblended ingredients remain or stick to the sides, use a spatula to scrape them down into the blended mixture and continue processing until thoroughly incorporated. The mixture will be a thick liquid.

3. Add the ice to the blender, close the lid, and process on the ice crush setting (or high speed) until the ingredients are smooth and the ice is thoroughly incorporated. The smoothie should have a thick, creamy consistency.

4. Serve immediately.

Variation Tip: Lemon is the lowest-carb citrus fruit, but other citrus can work in small quantities. Try freshly squeezed juice from half a lime or orange, or a quarter of a small grapefruit.

Per Serving: Macronutrients: 66% Fat, 30% Protein, 4% Carbs; Calories: 477; Total Fat: 35g; Protein: 36g; Total Carbs: 11g; Fiber: <1g; Net Carbs: 9g; Erythritol: 2g

Sweet Orange Cream Smoothie

Prep time: 5 minutes | **Yield:** 1 serving | High Fat

Freshly squeezed orange juice and cream come together in a classic pairing that's reminiscent of the famous creamy orange ice-cream bars. Unlike the dessert, this smoothie is low-carb and loaded with vitamin C.

½ **cup cold water**
½ **cup heavy (whipping) cream**
Juice of ½ medium orange
1 teaspoon vanilla extract

½ **teaspoon monkfruit erythritol blend**
 sweetener (or preferred sweetener)
1 cup crushed or cubed ice

1. In a blender, combine the water, heavy cream, orange juice, vanilla, and sweetener.

2. Secure the lid and process at high speed until the ingredients are smooth and well combined, 1 to 2 minutes. If unblended ingredients remain or stick to the sides, use a spatula to scrape them down into the blended mixture and continue processing until thoroughly incorporated. The mixture will be a thin liquid.

3. Add the ice to the blender, close the lid, and process on the ice crush setting (or high speed) until the ingredients are smooth and the ice is thoroughly incorporated into the mixture, 1 to 2 minutes. The smoothie should have a thick, creamy consistency.

4. Serve immediately.

Variation Tip: Add orange extract to boost the orange flavor without expanding the carb count.

Per Serving: Macronutrients: 86% Fat, 4% Protein, 10% Carbs; Calories: 437; Total Fat: 43g; Protein: 4g; Total Carbs: 10g; Fiber: <1g; Net Carbs: 10g

Yogurt Berry Protein Parfait Smoothie

Prep time: 5 minutes | **Yield:** 1 serving | High Protein

Looking for a protein boost without the hassle of cooking? Smoothie to the rescue! This one borrows the flavors of a classic breakfast parfait, complete with yogurt, berries, and hemp heart "granola."

1 cup cold water

½ cup plain full-fat Greek yogurt

1 tablespoon MCT oil

1 scoop whey protein isolate powder (or preferred protein powder)

½ teaspoon monkfruit erythritol blend sweetener (or preferred sweetener)

¼ cup fresh or frozen mixed berries

1 cup crushed or cubed ice (optional)

1 tablespoon hemp hearts, for garnish

1. In a blender, combine the water, Greek yogurt, MCT oil, protein powder, sweetener, and mixed berries.

2. Secure the lid and process at high speed until the ingredients are smooth and well combined, 1 to 2 minutes. If unblended ingredients remain or stick to the sides, use a spatula to scrape them down into the blended mixture and continue processing until thoroughly incorporated. The mixture will be a thick liquid.

3. If desired, add the ice to the blender, close the lid, and process on the ice crush setting (or high speed) until the ingredients are smooth and the ice is thoroughly incorporated into the mixture. The smoothie should have a thick, creamy consistency.

4. Pour the mixture into a serving glass and garnish with the hemp hearts. Enjoy immediately.

Per Serving: Macronutrients: 55% Fat, 37% Protein, 8% Carbs; Calories: 424; Total Fat: 26g; Protein: 39g; Total Carbs: 13g; Fiber: 1g; Net Carbs: 10g; Erythritol: 2g

Frozen Berries and Cream Protein Smoothie

Prep time: 5 minutes | **Yield:** 1 serving | High Protein

This refreshing recipe is delightful and nutritious—a healthy take on berries and cream. The protein shake is a great way to cool off after a demanding workout, and it makes a perfect breakfast or dessert on scorching-hot days.

¾ **cup cold water**

¼ **cup heavy (whipping) cream**

1 scoop whey protein isolate powder (or preferred protein powder)

½ **cup frozen mixed berries**

1 cup crushed or cubed ice (optional)

1. In a blender, combine the water, heavy cream, protein powder, and mixed berries.

2. Secure the lid and process at high speed until the ingredients are smooth and well combined, 1 to 2 minutes. If unblended ingredients remain or stick to the sides, use a spatula to scrape them down into the blended mixture and continue processing until thoroughly incorporated. The mixture will be a thick liquid.

3. If desired, add the ice to the blender, close the lid, and process on the ice crush setting (or high speed) until the ingredients are smooth and the ice is thoroughly incorporated. The smoothie should have a thick, creamy consistency.

4. Serve immediately.

Per Serving: Macronutrients: 59% Fat, 29% Protein, 12% Carbs; Calories: 367; Total Fat: 24g; Protein: 27g; Total Carbs: 12g; Fiber: 2g; Net Carbs: 10g

Net Carbs
12g

Mixed Berry Cinnamon Roll Smoothie

Prep time: 5 minutes | **Yield:** 1 serving | High Fat

Cinnamon rolls have a special place in my heart. I didn't think there was any improving on their perfection until I discovered a bakery selling them with berries swirling down the center. Pure genius! This smoothie is like that brilliant, sweet roll in a cup.

1 cup unsweetened almond milk (or preferred dairy-free milk)

2 tablespoons heavy (whipping) cream

1 teaspoon ground cinnamon

1 teaspoon erythritol brown sugar replacement (or preferred sweetener)

½ cup fresh or frozen mixed berries

2 tablespoons butter or ghee, melted and slightly cooled

1 cup crushed or cubed ice (optional)

1. In a blender, combine the almond milk, heavy cream, cinnamon, sweetener, and mixed berries.

2. Secure the lid and process at high speed until the ingredients are well combined, 1 to 2 minutes.

3. While the blender is running, slowly pour in the melted butter through the opening in the lid to prevent clumping. If unblended ingredients remain or stick to the sides, use a spatula to scrape them down into the blended mixture and continue processing until thoroughly incorporated. The mixture will be a thin liquid.

4. If desired, add the ice to the blender, close the lid, and process on the ice crush setting (or high speed) until the ingredients are smooth and the ice is thoroughly incorporated, 1 to 2 minutes. The smoothie should have a thick, creamy consistency.

5. Serve immediately.

Per Serving: Macronutrients: 85% Fat, 3% Protein, 12% Carbs; Calories: 382; Total Fat: 36g; Protein: 3g; Total Carbs: 19g; Fiber: 3g; Net Carbs: 12g; Erythritol: 4g

Raspberry Cottage Cheese Smoothie

Prep time: 5 minutes | **Yield:** 1 serving | High Fat, High Protein

Cottage cheese is an awesome high-protein smoothie add-in when you crave something besides protein powder or Greek yogurt. Its mellow flavor makes it a fantastic sidekick for a variety of ingredients, but tart, sweet raspberries lend themselves to a match made in heaven.

¾ **cup cold water**

¼ **cup heavy (whipping) cream**

1 **cup cottage cheese**

½ **cup fresh or frozen raspberries**

1 **cup crushed or cubed ice (optional)**

1. In a blender, combine the water, heavy cream, cottage cheese, and raspberries.

2. Secure the lid and process at high speed until the ingredients are smooth and well combined, 1 to 2 minutes. If unblended ingredients remain or stick to the sides, use a spatula to scrape them down into the blended mixture and continue processing until thoroughly incorporated. The mixture will be a thick liquid.

3. If desired, add the ice to the blender, close the lid, and process on the ice crush setting (or high speed) until the ingredients are smooth and the ice is thoroughly incorporated, 1 to 2 minutes. The smoothie should have a thick, creamy consistency.

4. Serve immediately.

Variation Tip: For a fun garnish, reserve some of the raspberries to top the smoothie, along with coconut flakes and seeds.

Per Serving: Macronutrients: 63% Fat, 24% Protein, 13% Carbs; Calories: 440; Total Fat: 31g; Protein: 26g; Total Carbs: 16g; Fiber: 4g; Net Carbs: 12g

Blueberry Lemon Cream Smoothie

Prep tim e: 5 minutes | **Yield:** 1 serving | High Fat

I first discovered the blueberry and lemon flavor combo while traveling with my mom. We visited a local farm stand that was selling double-scoop ice-cream cones. The most popular combo? One scoop blueberry, one scoop lemon. I have linked the two in matrimonial smoothie bliss ever since.

½ **cup cold water**

½ **cup heavy (whipping) cream**

Juice of ½ lemon

½ **cup fresh or frozen blueberries**

1 cup crushed or cubed ice (optional)

1. In a blender, combine the water, heavy cream, lemon juice, and blueberries.

2. Secure the lid and process at high speed until the ingredients are smooth and well combined, 1 to 2 minutes. If unblended ingredients remain or stick to the sides, use a spatula to scrape them down into the blended mixture and continue processing until thoroughly incorporated. The mixture will be a thick liquid.

3. If desired, add the ice to the blender, close the lid, and process on the ice crush setting (or high speed) until the ingredients are smooth and the ice is thoroughly incorporated. The smoothie should have a thick, creamy consistency.

4. Serve immediately.

Per Serving: Macronutrients: 86% Fat, 4% Protein, 10% Carbs; Calories: 452; Total Fat: 43g; Protein: 4g; Total Carbs: 16g; Fiber: 2g; Net Carbs: 14g

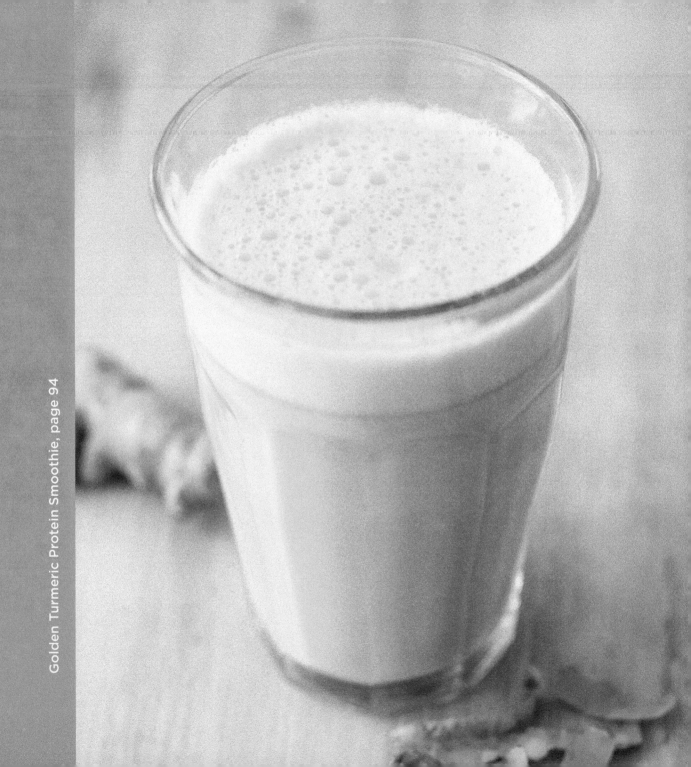

Golden Turmeric Protein Smoothie, page 94

CHAPTER 6

SAVORY

Sweetness isn't necessary for satisfied taste buds. Savory smoothies are a treat in their own right, and this chapter will prove it. The recipes in this chapter feature tastes that land outside the sweet spectrum, including umami, salty, sour, bitter, astringent, and pungent. Instead of sweets, you'll find a celebration of herbal flavors, innovative spice combinations, and loads of veggies. You'll see how to add savory ingredients to your smoothie-making bag of tricks without relying on sweeteners and sugary elements to disguise them.

Mascarpone Coffee Smoothie

Prep time: 5 minutes | **Yield:** 1 serving | High Fat, Super Low Carb

Skip those sweet coffee drinks and upgrade your java with some creamy mascarpone cheese. The luxurious velvety texture and savory flavor will provide you with a welcome respite from the typical sugar-loaded beverage.

1 cup unsweetened cold-brew coffee (or chilled black coffee)

¼ cup heavy (whipping) cream

2 tablespoons mascarpone cheese

1 cup crushed or cubed ice

1. In a blender, combine the coffee, heavy cream, and mascarpone.

2. Secure the lid and process at high speed until the ingredients are smooth and well combined, 1 to 2 minutes. If unblended ingredients remain or stick to the sides, use a spatula to scrape them down into the blended mixture and continue processing until thoroughly incorporated. The mixture will be a thick liquid.

3. Add the ice to the blender, close the lid, and process on the ice crush setting (or high speed) until the ingredients are smooth and the ice is thoroughly incorporated. The smoothie should have a thick, creamy consistency.

4. Serve immediately.

Per Serving: Macronutrients: 96% Fat, 3% Protein, 1% Carbs; Calories: 327; Total Fat: 35g; Protein: 3g; Total Carbs: 3g; Fiber: 0g; Net Carbs: 3g

Golden Turmeric Protein Smoothie

Prep time: 5 minutes | **Yield:** 1 serving | High Fat, High Protein, Super Low Carb

I may be a wee bit obsessed with blending turmeric in my smoothies. Of course, there are the countless health benefits, thanks to the anti-inflammatory and antioxidant properties of curcumin. But that cheerful orange hue has me adding it for a fun pop of color whenever I can.

1 cup unsweetened coconut milk beverage

1 scoop whey protein isolate powder (or preferred protein powder)

1 teaspoon turmeric powder

Pinch freshly ground black pepper

2 tablespoons coconut oil, melted

1 cup crushed or cubed ice

1. In a blender, combine the coconut milk beverage, protein powder, turmeric, and black pepper.

2. Secure the lid and process at high speed until the ingredients are well combined, 1 to 2 minutes.

3. While the blender is running, slowly pour in the melted coconut oil through the opening in the lid to prevent clumping. If unblended ingredients remain or stick to the sides, use a spatula to scrape them down into the blended mixture and continue processing until thoroughly incorporated. The mixture will be a thin liquid.

4. Add the ice to the blender, close the lid, and process on the ice crush setting (or high speed) until the ingredients are smooth and the ice is thoroughly incorporated. The smoothie should have a thick, fluffy consistency.

5. Serve immediately.

Per Serving: Macronutrients: 71% Fat, 24% Protein, 5% Carbs; Calories: 433; Total Fat: 34g; Protein: 26g; Total Carbs: 5g; Fiber: 1g; Net Carbs: 4g

Jicama Avocado Cilantro Lemon Smoothie

Prep time: 5 minutes | **Yield:** 1 serving | Super Low Carb

I adore jicama in both sweet and savory smoothies. Its mild, neutral flavor allows it to be partnered with just about anything. Rich in vitamins and minerals, this root vegetable adds a wonderful creamy texture when blended. Here, jicama unites with buttery avocado, bright lemon, and robust herbal cilantro.

1 cup cold water

Juice of ½ lemon

1 avocado, peeled, pitted, and cut into chunks

½ cup jicama, sliced

¼ cup chopped fresh cilantro

1 cup crushed or cubed ice (optional)

1. In a blender, combine the water, lemon juice, avocado, jicama, and cilantro.

2. Secure the lid and process at high speed until the ingredients are smooth and well combined, 1 to 2 minutes. If unblended ingredients remain or stick to the sides, use a spatula to scrape them down into the blended mixture and continue processing until thoroughly incorporated. The mixture will be a thick liquid.

3. If desired, add the ice to the blender, close the lid, and process on the ice crush setting (or high speed) until the ingredients are smooth and the ice is thoroughly incorporated, 1 to 2 minutes. The smoothie should have a thick, fluffy consistency.

4. Serve immediately.

Per Serving: Macronutrients: 79% Fat, 5% Protein, 16% Carbs; Calories: 240; Total Fat: 21g; Protein: 3g; Total Carbs: 15g; Fiber: 10g; Net Carbs: 5g

Buttery Radish Avocado Smoothie

Prep time: 5 minutes | **Yield:** 1 serving | High Fat, Super Low Carb

Buttery flavors are a surefire way to guarantee an unforgettable savory smoothie. The creamy texture and rich flavors of butter or ghee and avocado play well off the sharp, peppery radish.

1 cup cold water
Juice of ½ lemon
1 cup radishes, sliced
1 avocado, peeled, pitted, and cut
   into chunks

1 tablespoon butter or ghee, melted and
   slightly cooled
1 cup crushed or cubed ice (optional)

1. In a blender, combine the water, lemon juice, radishes, and avocado.

2. Secure the lid and process at high speed until the ingredients are well combined, 1 to 2 minutes.

3. While the blender is running, slowly pour in the melted butter through the opening in the lid to prevent clumping. If unblended ingredients remain or stick to the sides, use a spatula to scrape them down into the blended mixture and continue processing until thoroughly incorporated. The mixture will be a thick liquid.

4. If desired, add the ice to the blender, close the lid, and process on the ice crush setting (or high speed) until the ingredients are smooth and the ice is thoroughly incorporated, 1 to 2 minutes. The smoothie should have a thick, fluffy consistency.

5. Serve immediately.

Per Serving: Macronutrients: 84% Fat, 5% Protein, 11% Carbs; Calories: 353; Total Fat: 33g; Protein: 4g; Total Carbs: 17g; Fiber: 11g; Net Carbs: 6g

Creamy Kale Protein Smoothie

Prep time: 5 minutes | **Yield:** 1 serving | High Fat, High Protein, Super Low Carb

Kale is a staple in green smoothies for its wonderful earthy taste and nutritional value. This recipe is supercharged with vitamins, minerals, and phytonutrients; heavy cream ups the fat content for extra energy.

¾ **cup cold water**

¼ **cup heavy (whipping) cream**

Juice of ½ lemon

1 tablespoon extra-virgin olive oil

1 scoop whey protein isolate powder (or
  preferred protein powder)

½ **teaspoon ground ginger**

½ **teaspoon nutmeg**

2 cups kale, chopped, stemmed

1 cup crushed or cubed ice (optional)

1. In a blender, combine the water, heavy cream, lemon juice, olive oil, protein powder, ginger, nutmeg, and kale.

2. Secure the lid and process at high speed until the ingredients are smooth and well combined, 1 to 2 minutes. If unblended ingredients remain or stick to the sides, use a spatula to scrape them down into the blended mixture and continue processing until thoroughly incorporated. The mixture will be a thick liquid.

3. If desired, add the ice to the blender, close the lid, and process on the ice crush setting (or high speed) until the ingredients are smooth and the ice is thoroughly incorporated, 1 to 2 minutes. The smoothie should have a thick, creamy consistency.

4. Serve immediately.

Per Serving: Macronutrients: 71% Fat, 23% Protein, 6% Carbs; Calories: 481; Total Fat: 38g; Protein: 28g; Total Carbs: 8g; Fiber: 2g; Net Carbs: 6g

Herbal Dandelion Smoothie

Prep time: 5 minutes | **Yield:** 1 serving | Super Low Carb

Dandelions aren't just weeds in your lawn; they are nutritional powerhouses that deserve a spot in your smoothie arsenal—plus the whole plant's edible, from root to blossom! Here, the greens and root create a nutrient-dense herbal elixir that fights inflammation and oxidative stress.

1 cup brewed dandelion tea, chilled

Juice of ½ lemon

1 cup dandelion greens, cut into pieces

¼ cup hemp hearts

1 cup crushed or cubed ice (optional)

1. In a blender, combine the dandelion tea, lemon juice, dandelion greens, and hemp hearts.

2. Secure the lid and process at high speed until the ingredients are smooth and well combined, 1 to 2 minutes. If unblended ingredients remain or stick to the sides, use a spatula to scrape them down into the blended mixture and continue processing until thoroughly incorporated. The mixture will be a thick liquid.

3. If desired, add the ice to the blender, close the lid, and process on the ice crush setting (or high speed) until the ingredients are smooth and the ice is thoroughly incorporated, 1 to 2 minutes. The smoothie should have a thick, fluffy consistency.

4. Serve immediately.

Variation Tip: Consider experimenting with other herbal teas in place of dandelion. Ginger, rooibos, mint, and lemon balm teas are some excellent choices.

Per Serving: Macronutrients: 67% Fat, 23% Protein, 10% Carbs; Calories: 256; Total Fat: 19g; Protein: 15g; Total Carbs: 9g; Fiber: 3g; Net Carbs: 6g

Spiced Tomato Smoothie

Prep time: 5 minutes | **Yield:** 1 serving | Super Low Carb

Tomatoes are the unsung heroes of the smoothie world. These juicy fruits pair well with a variety of spices and flavors and flaunt high levels of vitamins, minerals, and antioxidants, like lycopene. Though they have a subtle, natural sweetness, they make an excellent addition to savory smoothies.

1 cup cold water

2 tablespoons MCT oil

½ teaspoon ground cinnamon

½ teaspoon ground nutmeg

½ teaspoon ground allspice

1 large tomato, cut into pieces

1 cup crushed or cubed ice (optional)

1. In a blender, combine the water, MCT oil, cinnamon, nutmeg, allspice, and tomato.

2. Secure the lid and process at high speed until the ingredients are smooth and well combined, 1 to 2 minutes. If unblended ingredients remain or stick to the sides, use a spatula to scrape them down into the blended mixture and continue processing until thoroughly incorporated. The mixture will be a thin liquid.

3. If desired, add the ice to the blender, close the lid, and process on the ice crush setting (or high speed) until the ingredients are smooth and the ice is thoroughly incorporated, 1 to 2 minutes. The smoothie should have a thick, fluffy consistency.

4. Serve immediately.

Per Serving: Macronutrients: 92% Fat, 3% Protein, 5% Carbs; Calories: 275; Total Fat: 28g; Protein: 2g; Total Carbs: 10g; Fiber: 3g; Net Carbs: 7g

Zucchini and Greens Protein Shake

Prep time: 5 minutes | **Yield:** 1 serving | High Fat, High Protein, Super Low Carb

With flavorful leafy greens, herbs, healthy fats, and nutrients galore, I like to think of green smoothies as sippable salads. Adding a zucchini to the mix results in a surprising creaminess when blended.

1 cup cold water

2 tablespoons MCT oil

1 scoop whey protein isolate powder (or preferred protein powder)

1 medium zucchini, cut into pieces

1 cup spinach, cut into pieces

1 cup kale, chopped, stemmed

½ cup arugula

¼ cup fresh mint

1. In a blender, combine the water, MCT oil, protein powder, zucchini, spinach, kale, arugula, and mint.

2. Secure the lid and process at high speed until the ingredients are smooth and well combined, 1 to 2 minutes. If unblended ingredients remain or stick to the sides, use a spatula to scrape them down into the blended mixture and continue processing until thoroughly incorporated. The smoothie should have a thick consistency.

3. Serve immediately.

Per Serving: Macronutrients: 67% Fat, 28% Protein, 5% Carbs; Calories: 417; Total Fat: 31g; Protein: 29g; Total Carbs: 11g; Fiber: 4g; Net Carbs: 7g

Cucumber Avocado Sesame Smoothie

Prep time: 5 minutes | **Yield:** 1 serving | High Fat, High Protein, Super Low Carb

Sesame seeds and sesame seed milk yield a delicate, nutty base for hydrating cucumber and earthy avocado. This recipe delivers a triple threat for your keto macros—low-carb, high-fat, and high-protein—plus it's packed with vitamins and minerals, especially potassium and magnesium electrolytes.

1 cup unsweetened sesame seed milk (or cold water)

2 tablespoons collagen hydrolysate powder

¼ cup sesame seeds

½ avocado, peeled, pitted, and cut into chunks

½ medium cucumber, cut into pieces

1 cup crushed or cubed ice (optional)

1. In a blender, combine the sesame seed milk, collagen powder, sesame seeds, avocado, and cucumber.

2. Secure the lid and process at high speed until the ingredients are smooth and well combined, 1 to 2 minutes. If unblended ingredients remain or stick to the sides, use a spatula to scrape them down into the blended mixture and continue processing until thoroughly incorporated. The mixture will be a thick liquid.

3. If desired, add the ice to the blender, close the lid, and process on the ice crush setting (or high speed) until the ingredients are smooth and the ice is thoroughly incorporated, 1 to 2 minutes. The smoothie should have a thick, fluffy consistency.

4. Serve immediately.

Variation Tip: Try adding chopped or crumbled dried nori for a subtle umami flavor.

Per Serving: Macronutrients: 63% Fat, 25% Protein, 12% Carbs; Calories: 444; Total Fat: 31g; Protein: 28g; Total Carbs: 20g; Fiber: 12g; Net Carbs: 8g

Virgin Bloody Mary Smoothie

Prep time: 5 minutes | **Yield:** 1 serving | Super Low Carb

Bloody Marys aren't just for brunch or happy hour! When you skip the booze, those trademark flavors make the perfect savory base for an anytime smoothie.

1 cup cold water

2 tablespoons tomato paste

1 teaspoon horseradish

1 teaspoon Worcestershire sauce

¼ teaspoon celery salt

1 medium celery stalk, cut into pieces

1 cup crushed or cubed ice (optional)

3 extra-large green olives, for garnish

2 ounces cheddar cheese, cubed,
  for garnish

1. In a blender, combine the water, tomato paste, horseradish, Worcestershire sauce, celery salt, and celery.

2. Secure the lid and process at high speed until the ingredients are smooth and well combined, 1 to 2 minutes. If unblended ingredients remain or stick to the sides, use a spatula to scrape them down into the blended mixture and continue processing until thoroughly incorporated. The mixture will be a thin liquid.

3. If desired, add the ice to the blender, close the lid, and process on the ice crush setting (or high speed) until the ingredients are smooth and the ice is thoroughly incorporated, 1 to 2 minutes. The smoothie should have a thick, fluffy consistency.

4. Pour the mixture into a serving glass and garnish with a cocktail pick skewering the olives and cheese cubes. Enjoy immediately.

Variation Tip: Tomato juice can replace the tomato paste and water for convenience, though the carb count will be slightly higher. You can also add bacon as a garnish.

Per Serving: Macronutrients: 67% Fat, 20% Protein, 13% Carbs; Calories: 297; Total Fat: 22g; Protein: 15g; Total Carbs: 12g; Fiber: 3g; Net Carbs: 9g

Red Bell Pepper and Basil Protein Smoothie

Prep time: 5 minutes | **Yield:** 1 serving | High Fat, High Protein

Bell peppers make an outstanding addition to smoothies. Though green bell peppers are lowest in carbs, the red variety delivers the biggest nutritional bang. Red bell peppers are harvested later, allowing more time to ripen, which produces higher vitamin C, beta-carotene, and potassium levels.

1 cup unsweetened almond milk (or preferred dairy-free milk)

2 tablespoons avocado oil (or preferred oil)

1 scoop whey protein isolate powder (or preferred protein powder)

1 red bell pepper, stemmed and seeds removed, cut into pieces

½ cup chopped fresh basil

1 cup crushed or cubed ice (optional)

1. In a blender, combine the almond milk, avocado oil, protein powder, bell pepper, and basil.

2. Secure the lid and process at high speed until the ingredients are smooth and well combined, 1 to 2 minutes. If unblended ingredients remain or stick to the sides, use a spatula to scrape them down into the blended mixture and continue processing until thoroughly incorporated. The mixture will be a thin liquid.

3. If desired, add the ice to the blender, close the lid, and process on the ice crush setting (or high speed) until the ingredients are smooth and the ice is thoroughly incorporated, 1 to 2 minutes. The smoothie should have a thick, fluffy consistency.

4. Serve immediately.

Per Serving: Macronutrients: 65% Fat, 25% Protein, 10% Carbs; Calories: 443; Total Fat: 32g; Protein: 28g; Total Carbs: 13g; Fiber: 3g; Net Carbs: 10g

Garlic Lemon Broccoli and Almond Smoothie

Prep time: 5 minutes | **Yield:** 1 serving

Many broccoli smoothie recipes use sugary fruits and syrups to mask its earthy, green taste. This one celebrates the unique herbaceous flavor, using complementary ingredients that highlight the veggie rather than disguising it.

1 cup unsweetened almond milk (or preferred dairy-free milk)

Juice of ½ lemon

2 tablespoons unsweetened almond butter

1 garlic clove, crushed

1 cup chopped or riced frozen broccoli

1. In a blender, combine the almond milk, lemon juice, almond butter, garlic, and broccoli.

2. Secure the lid and process at high speed until the ingredients are smooth and well combined, 1 to 2 minutes. If unblended ingredients remain or stick to the sides, use a spatula to scrape them down into the blended mixture and continue processing until thoroughly incorporated. The smoothie should have a thick consistency.

3. Serve immediately.

Per Serving: Macronutrients: 65% Fat, 17% Protein, 18% Carbs; Calories: 278; Total Fat: 20g; Protein: 12g; Total Carbs: 19g; Fiber: 9g; Net Carbs: 10g

Carrot Ginger Turmeric Smoothie

Prep time: 5 minutes | **Yield:** 1 serving | High Fat

This immune-boosting breakfast will help sustain your energy all morning long. It'll also reward your taste buds and supply the nutritional components that bolster your body's natural defenses against chronic disease and infection.

1 cup unsweetened coconut milk beverage

2 tablespoons avocado oil (or extra-virgin olive oil)

1 teaspoon turmeric powder

1 teaspoon ground ginger

Pinch freshly ground black pepper

1 cup chopped fresh or frozen carrots

1 cup crushed or cubed ice (optional)

1. In a blender, combine the coconut milk beverage, avocado oil, turmeric, ginger, black pepper, and carrots.

2. Secure the lid and process at high speed until the ingredients are smooth and well combined, 1 to 2 minutes. If unblended ingredients remain or stick to the sides, use a spatula to scrape them down into the blended mixture and continue processing until thoroughly incorporated. The mixture will be a thick liquid.

3. If desired, add the ice to the blender, close the lid, and process on the ice crush setting (or high speed) until the ingredients are smooth and the ice is thoroughly incorporated, 1 to 2 minutes. The smoothie should have a thick, fluffy consistency.

4. Serve immediately.

Per Serving: Macronutrients: 83% Fat, 3% Protein, 14% Carbs; Calories: 359; Total Fat: 33g; Protein: 3g; Total Carbs: 17g; Fiber: 5g; Net Carbs: 12g

Spiced Cauliflower Yogurt Smoothie

Prep time: 5 minutes | **Yield:** 1 serving | High Protein

This creamy smoothie boasts the anti-inflammatory properties of cinnamon, ginger, and turmeric with the high-protein content of Greek yogurt. Cauliflower adds bulk and substance as well as fiber, vitamin C, and potassium.

1 cup unsweetened coconut milk beverage (or preferred dairy-free milk)

¾ cup plain full-fat Greek yogurt

1 teaspoon ground cinnamon

½ teaspoon ground ginger

½ teaspoon ground turmeric

Pinch freshly ground black pepper

1 tablespoon coconut oil, melted and slightly cooled

1½ cups chopped or riced frozen cauliflower

1. In a blender, combine the coconut milk beverage, yogurt, cinnamon, ginger, turmeric, and black pepper. Secure the lid and process at high speed until the ingredients are well combined, 1 to 2 minutes.

2. While the blender is running, slowly pour in the melted coconut oil through the opening in the lid to prevent clumping. If unblended ingredients remain or stick to the sides, use a spatula to scrape them down into the blended mixture and continue processing until thoroughly incorporated. The smoothie should have a thick, fluffy consistency.

3. Add the frozen cauliflower to the blender, close the lid, and process on the ice crush setting (or high speed) until the ingredients are smooth and the cauliflower is thoroughly incorporated, 1 to 2 minutes. Serve immediately.

Per Serving: Macronutrients: 61% Fat, 22% Protein, 17% Carbs; Calories: 381; Total Fat: 26g; Protein: 21g; Total Carbs: 19g; Fiber: 6g; Net Carbs: 13g

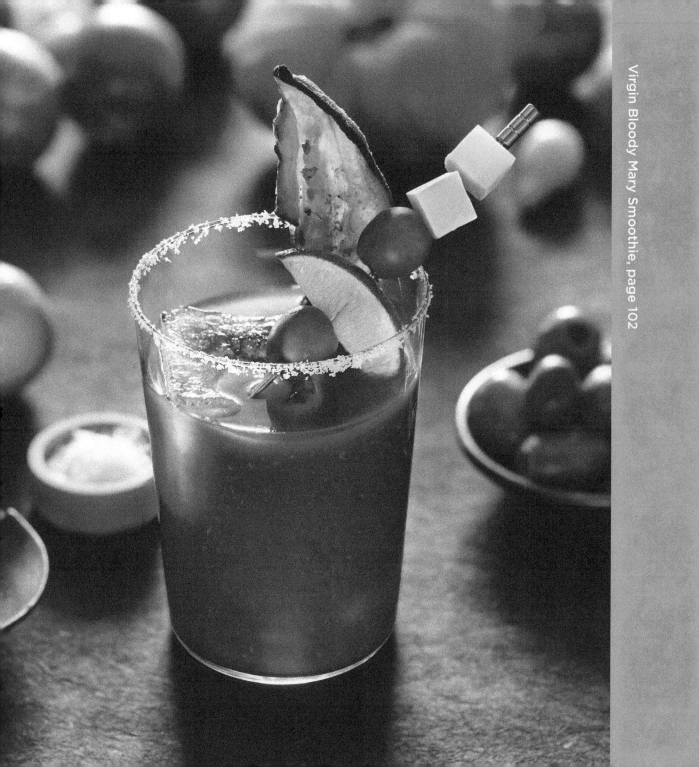

Virgin Bloody Mary Smoothie, page 102

MEASUREMENT CONVERSIONS

VOLUME EQUIVALENTS	U.S. STANDARD	U.S. STANDARD (OUNCES)	METRIC (APPROXIMATE)
LIQUID	2 tablespoons	1 fl. oz.	30 mL
	¼ cup	2 fl. oz.	60 mL
	½ cup	4 fl. oz.	120 mL
	1 cup	8 fl. oz.	240 mL
	1½ cups	12 fl. oz.	355 mL
	2 cups or 1 pint	16 fl. oz.	475 mL
	4 cups or 1 quart	32 fl. oz.	1 L
	1 gallon	128 fl. oz.	4 L
DRY	⅛ teaspoon	—	0.5 mL
	¼ teaspoon	—	1 mL
	½ teaspoon	—	2 mL
	¾ teaspoon	—	4 mL
	1 teaspoon	—	5 mL
	1 tablespoon	—	15 mL
	¼ cup	—	59 mL
	⅓ cup	—	79 mL
	½ cup	—	118 mL
	⅔ cup	—	156 mL
	¾ cup	—	177 mL
	1 cup	—	235 mL
	2 cups or 1 pint	—	475 mL
	3 cups	—	700 mL
	4 cups or 1 quart	—	1 L
	½ gallon	—	2 L
	1 gallon	—	4 L

OVEN TEMPERATURES

FAHRENHEIT	CELSIUS (APPROXIMATE)
250°F	120°C
300°F	150°C
325°F	165°C
350°F	180°C
375°F	190°C
400°F	200°C
425°F	220°C
450°F	230°C

WEIGHT EQUIVALENTS

U.S. STANDARD	METRIC (APPROXIMATE)
½ ounce	15 g
1 ounce	30 g
2 ounces	60 g
4 ounces	115 g
8 ounces	225 g
12 ounces	340 g
16 ounces or 1 pound	455 g

INDEX

Acknowledgments

There are lots of people I'd like to thank for helping make this book a reality, but foremost is my editor, Anna Pulley, for making this such an enjoyable process. You're the real MVP! Yoshita Jain, for thinking of me for this project. And to the entire team at Callisto Media, thank you for being such a pleasure to work with.

Sebina, for brainstorming fun recipes and ingredient combinations to include in this cookbook. Your Chocolate Coconut Cream Smoothie (page 60) is one of my faves!

Felix, for being such a committed taste tester. You're a more adventurous eater than you get credit for, bud.

Bradley, for supporting all my wild ideas, including temporarily converting our kitchen into a full-blown smoothie assembly line.

Grandma Bev and Scottie, for your overwhelming positivity and support of my cookbooks.

And last but not least, Mom, Tiff, and Trev, for celebrating all my milestones, big and small. You guys are always there to cheer me on, and it means the world to me.

About the Author

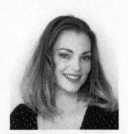

Tasha Metcalf is a writer, nutritionist, recipe developer, and founder of the wildly popular website Ketogasm.com. She creates healthy, down-to-earth recipes for low-carb and keto dietary patterns using accessible ingredients and unfussy techniques. Tasha also teaches the well-known Hello Keto course and online nutrition workshops. She lives in Tacoma, Washington, with her partner, Bradley, and their two amazing kiddos.